Intermittent Fasting for Women Over 50

The Complete Guide to Boost Your Metabolism, Gain Energy, Improve Weight Loss & Balanced Hormones. Detox Your Body and Promote Longevity After 50 with Autophagy.

By

dr. Michael Jason Young

Under no circumstances will any legal responsibility or blame be held against the publisher for any reparation, damages, or monetary loss due to the information herein, either directly or indirectly.

Respective authors own all copyrights not held by the publisher.

The information herein is offered for informational purposes solely and is universal as so. The presentation of the information is without contract or any type of guarantee assurance.

The trademarks that are used are without any consent, and the publication of the trademark is without permission or backing by the trademark owner. All trademarks and brands within this book are for clarifying purposes only and are the owned by the owners themselves, not affiliated with this document.

Table of Contents

Introduction

Intermittent Fasting is a concept that refers to a period of time where you don't eat. Fasting is a term that almost everyone is comfortable with. The causes for Fasting differ from one party to the next. It is a sacred ritual for some; they lack food in order to devote themselves to meditation. Others have little reason; they just don't have enough food. People used to go out to the countryside to farm and eat only while they were resting.

But intermittent Fasting is not just one of the Fasting mentioned above methods. It is a choice, not a faith tradition, nor is it motivated by a shortage of time or food. It's better characterized as a dietary plan that switches between cycles of eating and cycles of Fasting, each spanning a certain length of time. The 16:8 method, for instance, has a 16-hour fast followed by an 8-hour feeding time. It's important to note that this is not a diet but more an eating routine. There is little emphasis on the things you should consume, but there is more importance on where you should eat them. Would this imply that you are free to consume whatever you want? Regrettably, the response is no. You can bring out of existence what you put in, just like everything else. Clean eating is one of the three components of the fat-burning trifecta. Would this suggest you'll have to eat chicken and broccoli for the rest of your life? No way, no how. We are all humans and the key to living life to the fullest, but as you know, balance is the key.

It's crucial to understand that intermittent Fasting isn't a one-off initiative that can continue for a while before dissipating, as most weight-loss plans do. It has been famous for several years which has been around for a long time (even if you are discovering it just now). It is currently one of the most common health and wellness phenomena in the world. A number of wellness and lifestyle professionals endorse it. So if you're an aging woman who wants to discover her secret to longevity, intermittent Fasting is the go-to for you.

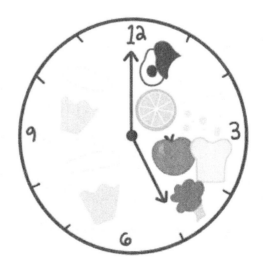

Chapter 1: Introduction to Intermittent Fasting

We are all aware that we ought to consume food more healthily. We all recognize that we can restrict our intake of soda, juice, refined foods, and sugars. Even if we are aware of these facts, it does not imply that they are simple to apply.

According to a new Psychology, Today diet and fitness poll, 52 percent of westerners feel it is simpler to work out their taxes than to figure out how to live healthily. Many individuals are frustrated with the new tax code, which ensures that even more individuals are having difficulty finding out how to eat a healthy diet. We exist in a world where obesity is a major problem. Obesity affects more than a portion of the world's populace, and even more, they are overweight. These figures, however, do not include a full view. Two out of every three adults are overweight or obese, which means that most individuals would fall under this group.

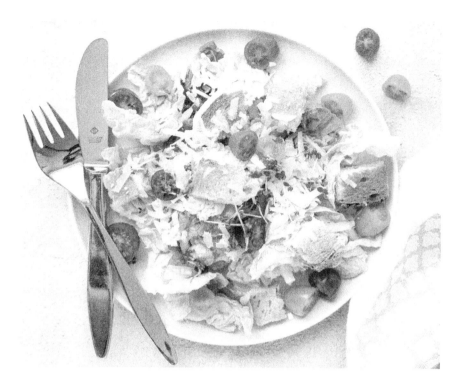

Why are these figures so depressing? A variety of causes may cause obesity. The traditional western diet is a major contributor. As we transitioned from a country that relies on food from small farmers to one that mass-produces most of our food, the consistency of our diets has deteriorated dramatically. Since food is now so easily accessible, we have expanded our intake due to this transformation. Furthermore, many widely obtainable and comfortable foods are rich in fat, carbohydrates, and calories. Any of these factors lead to weight gain. The quality of diet and the volume we consume has changed dramatically, from the sugary foods we encounter in the lunchroom and all of the fast-food stores that surround us. Obesity is too common in our society that we will actually consume fatty things indefinitely.

The first thing we can consider is the amount of food we consume. The amount of calories required by each person is different. Genetics, fitness level, physical wellbeing, height, age, and gender are all factors to consider. Nevertheless, the daily calorie intake recommended on food labels is about 2000 calories. For all those who lead sedentary lives, this figure is still very strong. When you go out to dinner, you will easily consume 2000 calories or more in one sitting. Although dining out soon drives us over our calorie thresholds, eating at home allows us to consume more. It's crucial to understand how to consume just what we need to survive, rather than consuming because something feels nice or because we're bored, lazy, or sad. It's also important to consider what time of day we feed. The majority of Americans lead hectic lives and do not have time to settle down and enjoy a very healthy meal. Instead, they feed on the move, normally at an unhealthy establishment or late at night, while their metabolic rates are sluggish. Furthermore, many Westerners watch tv while lying on the sofa consuming fatty snack products. When food is plentiful, we like to consume it incessantly.

It's important to understand how to take the right measures to limit how much food we consume each day. It's simple to be tempted by foods that are readily accessible. However, if you wish to restore your fitness and remain in shape, you must abandon the traditional American diet to favor something healthy and more beneficial to you.

1.1 What is Intermittent Fasting?

When you hear the word "fasting," you can conjure up images of people who abstain from eating for weeks on end for religious purposes. You might believe eating is unhealthy or that you won't be able to do it because you are addicted to food. On the other hand, intermittent Fasting is distinct from religious Fasting, beyond the fact that they share some similar concepts. Intermittent Fasting entails limiting calorie consumption at specific times during the day or not consuming too much on certain days. Your body always receives the nutrition it needs, so you consume fewer calories, making weight loss simpler. Later in the novel, several of the many forms of intermittent Fasting would be covered.

This diet is beneficial because it effectively reduces the amount of fat in your body as well as the number of calories you consume. Since you're limiting the amount of time you may consume or decreasing the calorie consumption for some days of the week, it's far better to and the total calorie intake.

You will still decide how long you want to go on an intermittent fast for. Some individuals do so for a month or so, while some make it a part of their daily routine and stay with it for the long haul. Let's aim for an eating pattern that would make it possible to shed weight and become happier now that we've looked at how the American diet is getting us overweight. This chapter will explain the basics of intermittent Fasting so you can see if it's right for you. Dieters who practice intermittent fasting alternate between times when they can eat and intervals where they are required to wait. This diet does not specify which foods you should consume but rather when you can eat them. Of necessity, eating healthy things for you and safe is preferable if you want to shed pounds or improve your fitness. On the other hand, intermittent Fasting does not specify which things you should and cannot consume.

Intermittent Fasting may be done in various ways, but they both divide the day or week through feeding and fasting times. You may be shocked to learn that most of us still fast when sleeping every day. You would be able to stretch the quick natural period a little further. You might opt to miss breakfast and eat your first meal at noon and your last meal at 8 p.m., for example. Intermittent Fasting is a concept used to describe this form of eating. This procedure requires you to fast for sixteen hours per day and then just feed for eight hours. When it comes to intermittent Fasting, this process, also known as the 16/8 method, is among the most common. Intermittent Fasting is probably better than you thought, despite what you might be hearing right now. It takes very little preparation, and many people who have tried this diet say that they feel healthier and have more stamina when fasting. You may experience some hunger at first, but it won't be long until your body adjusts and becomes used to it.

The most important thing to note is that you are not able to feed during the fasting time. You should choose to consume beverages to stay hydrated. Tea, coffee, water, as well as other non-caloric drinks are among the choices. Few versions of this fast allow for a small amount of food during Fasting, although the majority do not.

And, as long as the replacement does not include calories, it is usually good to take one on this fast.

The next concern you may have is whether you should even think about fasting in the first place. Humans have practiced fasting for thousands of years. They accomplished this because they were hungry and couldn't find something more to consume. Then there were the days that people fasted for social purposes. Fasting is needed in many religions, including Buddhism, Christianity, and Islam. When you are ill, it is often normal to fast.

While Fasting may have a different meaning, there really is nothing inherently abnormal about it. In reality, our bodies are well-prepared to go without food for extended periods of time. When we go on a high, several internal processes shift. This allows our bodies to act normally during times of drought. Fasting causes a substantial decrease in insulin levels, sugar levels, and a sharp increase in the human growth hormone. Although this was first used to help people lose weight as the food was unavailable, it is still used to lower cholesterol. Fasting makes fat burning easy, faster, and more efficient.

Some people like to fast to improve their stamina. This form of Fasting is beneficial for a variety of chronic health diseases. Intermittent Fasting can even help you live longer, according to some research. Intermittent Fasting has been shown to increase the lifetime of rodents in studies. Fasting has since been shown to guard against illnesses including Alzheimer's, cancer, type 2 diabetes, and cardiac failure in other studies. There are even many who want to fast intermittently because it is more comfortable for their lifestyle. Fasting can be a great way to save time and money. The fewer foods you have to prepare, for example, the easier your life can get.

1.2   Intermittent Fasting Vs. Other Forms of Fasting

Intermittent Fasting is the ritual of planning your meals in advance to ensure that the body gets the maximum benefit from them. Intermittent Fasting is an easy, sensible, and healthy form of eating that encourages weight reduction rather than halving your calorie consumption, robbing yourself of all your favorite foods, or jumping into the latest diet fad. Intermittent Fasting may be approached in various ways, although it is essentially characterized as a particular eating pattern.

Instead of adjusting what you consume, this approach involves altering what you consume.

When you first start intermittent Fasting, you'll still maintain your calorie consumption the same, except instead of eating smaller meals during the day, you'll consume larger meals over a shorter period of time. Instead of consuming three or four servings a day, you might consume one big meal at 11 a.m., then another major meal at 6 p.m., and no meals before 11 a.m. than 6 p.m., and no meals after 6 p.m. before 11 a.m. the very next day. This is just one form of intermittent Fasting; some may be covered in later chapters of this book. However, you must first comprehend that this technique works. Most bodybuilders, runners, and exercise gurus use intermittent Fasting to maintain their muscle mass up and their body fat percentage down. It's a straightforward approach that helps you consume the foods you like while also encouraging weight loss and muscle growth. Intermittent Fasting may be done over a brief or long time, but the strongest effects come from incorporating it into everyday routine.

While the word "fasting" may conjure up images of starvation in the mind of the common citizen, intermittent Fasting is not the same as starvation. We'll go through the two stages of digestion in the body, the fed condition, and the fasting state, to explain the principles behind active intermittent Fasting. The body is in what is

considered the "fed zone" for three to five hours after consuming a meal. Insulin levels rise in the fed state to help you eat and digest your food. It is very challenging for your body to burn fat while your insulin levels are strong. Insulin is the hormone released by the pancreas that helps to control blood glucose levels. Insulin is essentially a storage hormone, despite its regulatory role. Insulin prevents weight reduction because it causes the body to burn your diet for energy instead of your fat reserves when levels are large.

Your system will quit absorbing the food after three to five hours, and you are still in the post-absorptive stage. The post-absorptive condition will continue for up to 12 hours. Your body reaches the fasted condition during this time gap. Your blood sugars are poor at this stage because your body has totally consumed your food, rendering your stored fat highly available for burning.

When you're fasting, the body doesn't have many calories to use for energy, so it burns accumulated fat instead. Intermittent Fasting helps the body achieve a higher fat-burning level than you can for a typical three-meal-per-day feeding schedule. This consideration alone explains why many people see the rapid success of intermittent Fasting without changing their workout, schedules, eating

habits, or what they consume. They're clearly altering their eating habits in terms of pacing and pattern. It, of course, takes a little while to get into the groove of things when you start an intermittent fasting program. Don't be disheartened! If you have a drag, just get back into the intermittent fasting routine as soon as you are able. Avoid criticizing or feeling bad for yourself. Negative body talk can only delay a return to your old habits. Creating a lifestyle shift requires commitment, and no one requires you to do things right the first time. Intermittent Fasting can require some becoming used to if you aren't used to going without food for lengthy stretches of time. You'll get the grasp of it in no period if you pick the best strategy for you, keep centered, and stay confident.

Unlike several other diet schemes, the intermittent fast is one that would really work for you. It makes use of the body and how it acts to assist you in losing weight. When you learn of Fasting, it's simple to get nervous. You will believe that going without food for days or weeks would be too difficult for you (and who has the stamina to go without nutrition for that long even though they try to lose weight) and that it would be too difficult for you.

Intermittent Fasting isn't as easy as you would think. Fasting for weeks at a time is not only difficult, but it is also unhealthy for the body. If you fast for an extended period of time, your body can also go into starvation mode. It is assumed that you are in a period where you are not eating anything because your body can try to conserve calories to help you retain fat content for as long as humanly possible. This suggests you're not only starving, but you're still skipping out on weight loss.

You don't need to be concerned with how this sporadic fast would operate in a malnutrition situation. The intermittent fast is successful since you are not fasting for such a long time that the body enters hunger mode and avoids losing weight. Instead, it would help the fast last just well enough for your metabolism to pick up the pace. When you go for a few hours without food (generally no more than 24 hrs) on an erratic fast, you'll notice that your body doesn't go into survival mode right away. Instead, it will eat whatever calories are available. If you ate the recommended amount of calories for the day, your body would return to burning fat accumulated in your body as food. As a result, when you implement an intermittent fasting schedule, the body is forced to burn additional fat without investing in any more effort.

Here are a few fast performance tips:

1. First and foremost, you do not wait to see instant benefits from your current lifestyle. Instead, you'll need to stick to the procedure for at least 30 days before you can evaluate the outcome correctly.

2. Second, bear in mind that the consistency of the food you eat also counts since a few fast-food meals will erase all of your diligent work.

3. Finally, you can include a light workout regimen on fast days and a more conventional routine on full-calorie days with better performance.

Intermittent Fasting comes in a variety of forms. You may select from a few different forms of intermittent Fasting to try. These fasts may all be beneficial, and which one is best for you can be determined by your personal interests, schedule, and way of life. Fasting may be done in a variety of ways, including:

- The 5:2 diet needs you to fast two days a week. You are only permitted to consume 500-600 calories per day during those days

- The 16/8 system requires you to fast for 16 hours a day and feed for the remaining 8 hours. You should feed either from midday to 8 p.m. or from 10 a.m. to 6 p.m. You can choose any eight-hour timeframe that you pick.

- Eat-Stop-Eat: Once or twice a week, you can go without food from dinner one day to dinner the next. This encourages you to fast for 24 hours while also allowing you to feed on each of the days you are fasting.

There really are, of course, variants on the three mentioned above. Under this diet, certain individuals, for example, opt to restrict their hours even more and just feed for four hours and abstain for twenty. The 16/8 approach is used by many folks who go on such fasts because it is the simplest to adhere to and produces excellent performance. Intermittent Fasting is an easy and efficient way to lose weight. It allows you to consume fewer calories and burn additional calories and fat than you can on a regular diet.

1.3 Myths About Intermittent Fasting

There are several theories and concerns that you might have heard from other people or women, to be specific, and it's critical to dispel them because these stereotypes make people fearful of Fasting because of dogmas they've been taught over the past 15 years or so. But it's critical

to debunk these theories, so here are a few myths cleared for you.

Myth: Fasting causes overeating

You'll be hungry after a short. Many people believe that this hunger would lead to bingeing. The proof, on the other hand, refutes this concern. Ad libitum feeding refers to the process of allowing participants to consume as much as they like during a fasting study. They feed to their hearts' content and still stay slim. In reality, many intermittent fasting protocols would cause you to consume fewer rather than more. As a result of the moderate calorie limit, you'll lose weight gradually without slowing down your metabolism.

Myth: Intermittent Fasting reduces metabolic rates

We've been advised that eating often boosts our metabolism. This isn't entirely true, but intermittent Fasting might have had the contrary effect during a suitable time frame. Intermittent Fasting has been shown in studies to improve metabolism by 3.6-14 percent, including the reality that our calories will come from various sources, which is the deciding factor of whether or not we lose weight.

Myth: If you skip breakfast, you'll gain weight

Breakfast is sometimes misunderstood as the essential nutrition of the day. Breakfast deprivation is generally thought to trigger increased appetite, cravings, and

excess weight. There was no weight disparity between those who consumed breakfast and those who didn't in a 16-week survey of 283 people who were overweight or obese. As a result, while there might be some human variability, breakfast does not have a significant impact on your weight. According to specific reports, people who lose weight over time prefer to skip breakfast. Furthermore, adolescents and teens who consume breakfast have higher academic performance. As a result, it's essential to give attention to the unique requirements. Some people benefit from breakfast, and others will go without it without repercussions.

Myth: intermittent Fasting induces muscle destruction

This is accurate if you do it incorrectly, but if performed properly, you would not lose muscle as long as you consume sufficient protein during a 24-hour cycle or a week. Intermittent Fasting can never induce muscle weakness or atrophy as long as you consume enough and pair it with weight exercise and dieting. This is how you burn the glycogen stocks in the muscles, which causes endogenous fats to be transformed into ketone particles like Acetone, which acts as power. You will lose muscle mass as your body burns protein, but you must remember that as long as you consume sufficient food with enough fats in your

system, you will not have to sacrifice muscle mass.

Myth: When fasting, you cannot drink water

Many spiritual fasts, such as Ramadan Fasting, limit all water and food. Unrelated to this, a host of reports have emerged claiming that no-water fasts are beneficial to one's fitness. Due to the diuretic impact of Fasting, limiting water can contribute to a serious deficiency. That's why, when supervising patients on surgical fasts, doctors pay particular attention to fluid consumption. Electrolytes, including sodium and potassium, which are also vigorously peed out during Fasting, are often monitored by doctors. What's the implication? Throughout a fast, drink plenty of water and take potassium and sodium supplements if the fast lasts more than 13 or 14 hours.

Myth: Intermittent Fasting causes testosterone levels to drop

This is entirely untrue, much like the muscle failure and metabolism suppression fallacy, except it's a bit more complex since many experiments have found that

testosterone levels decrease following extended Fasting but then rise to much higher levels after weeks of Fasting. On the other hand, Fasting raises testosterone levels during regular fasting cycles, especially those lasting less than 24 hours. Thus, tests have shown that if you monitor people's testosterone levels at night while they are well fed , and then check their testosterone levels the next morning when they are fasting, the testosterone levels in the fasting group rise around 20- 30 times more than in the "fed" study. Fasting is a source of physical stress, which is why testosterone levels rise through extended Fasting. Stress raises cortisol levels, which aid testosterone production and growth hormone output, which help retain muscle mass.

Myth: Intermittent Fasting is harmful to women's health

This is something most women are concerned about. Experts, on the other hand, have differing viewpoints. However, pre-menopausal women can experience hormone adjustments during Intermittent Fasting, although this is more common during prolonged Fasting. The explanation why intermittent Fasting can be challenging for women is because people are more vulnerable to stress, and Fasting is a body source of stress that some women cannot manage. However, many other ladies fast for 20 hours a day and have no problems with their hormone balance. To summarise, this is dependent on the woman's genetic disposition since some women are more adaptable to the demands of intermittent Fasting, while others cannot. As a result, everything is dependent on you. You should achieve that if every day is going well for you - you're gaining weight, feeling energized, and there are no hormone issues or shifts. For those that feel some kind of disturbance, it is advised that you start small and progressively expand the duration of your intermittent Fasting for your body to respond to the adjustments progressively.

Myth: lack of energy is caused by fasting

Food is a source of energy. Would your energy levels drop if you don't have them? Yes, eventually. When you restrict intermittently, the cells switch to a certain pool of energy: body fat. There's enough of it to go around. That's right. Even a thin individual (e.g., 150 pounds with 10% body fat) has significant fat reserves to meet energy demands when fasting. Fifteen pounds of fat equals over 60,000 calories of energy if you do the calculations. In reality, many people claim that exercising when fasted gives them more power. After a big meal, blood is drawn away from tissues and digestive organs, making sense.

Myth: If you eat a lot, you'll lose weight

When it comes to weight loss, intermittent Fasting is highly beneficial. To see how you're gaining weight, you don't have to start measuring calories. What you have to do is stay away from processed goods and eat whole foods instead. If you're determined to lose weight quickly, combining extended Fasting with a ketogenic diet can provide incredible results. (Write a review of this book, and you will receive a fantastic KETO Cookbook for Women over 50 with over 650 recipes. Read the instructions at the end of this book).

Myth: Eating often can lead to weight loss

Eating more often has little impact on weight reduction because it does not increase metabolism. Indeed, a survey of 16 obese people showed no differences in weight, fat reduction, or appetite whether they ate three or six meals per day. Some people say that consuming makes it difficult to maintain a balanced diet. If you think exercising more often makes it possible for you to consume fewer calories and less fast food, go ahead and do so.

Myth: It Doesn't Get Rid of Toxins

That's so untrue. One of the great things about calorie restriction is how it helps the body becoming a well-oiled machine by reducing toxic load. Autophagy, the mechanism by which your cells remove waste materials, is triggered while fasting.

When you abstain, you are filtering out the "junk" via autophagy. This mechanism seems essential for the longevity of all of your body's cells and has been related to a longer lifespan. The best thing is that there's also an herbal supplement to help you get the most out of your detox, disinfect your cells, and reap the rewards of intermittent Fasting. It comes in the shape of activated charcoal, another fad-turned-lifestyle option. If you're new to Fasting, it's especially necessary to use items that help your body's waste disposal mechanism by capturing and escorting contaminants out. This is because the body will not tolerate the chemicals emitted into your system from your body fat when you first begin fasting.

1.4 Frequently Asked Questions About Intermittent Fasting

Intermittent Fasting can raise several questions in your mind. You want to be sure you're doing it correctly and that you'll be happy to reap all of the advantages that this diet plan promises. This chapter would go further into intermittent Fasting and what you need to do to make it work for you.

Is there someone who does not need to fast?

Intermittent Fasting is generally considered healthy for most individuals. It's a successful diet plan that emphasizes balanced food and having the calories and vitamins your body requires while limiting the amount of time you will eat. However, certain people should avoid going on an erratic high. This is primarily due to concerns that they would not be able to provide the nutrients they need. This kind of fast cannot be undertaken if you are underweight. Since you need to consume foods during the day to help your infant while pregnant or nursing, intermittent Fasting is not a choice for you.

If I fast, will I go into starvation mode?

There are also misconceptions about Fasting. These misconceptions are circulated so often that they are mistaken for facts. Any of the fasting theories you might be aware of are:

- You can go hungry if you are fasting.

- You will be hungry if you are fasting.

Fasting causes you to overeat until the fast is done, and it causes you to lose muscle tone. This has been debunked numerous times. Instead of heading into starvation mode, the body can begin to eat the excess fat it has accumulated. This will assist you in losing stubborn belly fat and being healthy, mainly if you have been eating sugar for a number of years.

What are some of the negative consequences of Fasting?

When you're on a fast, you'll have to live with a few side effects. These are normally very easy, and they will go away until your body has adjusted to the diet and has developed good eating habits. The below are some of the possible side effects:

- Constipation is a frequent side effect of this medication. If you're suffering from constipation, certain laxatives may help relieve the pain and nausea.

- Headaches: Some individuals get migraines when they first begin a fast, but they usually go away after a few days. Eating a little extra salt each day is a healthy way to cope with this.

- Stomach Pain: If the belly is gurgling, sparkling water is a safe option.

How can I deal with hunger?

The most crucial thing to remember is that hunger is a

temporary state. Most people fear that their hunger will intensify until it becomes unbearable, but this is seldom the case. Hunger manifests itself in bursts. Ignoring it and consuming some tea, coffee, or green tea will help you deal with your appetite.

Would my Fasting cause me to lose muscle?

This is a typical misunderstanding that many people have while contemplating an intermittent long. The body would first break down glycogen into glucose during fasting cycles so that it can be used for energy. When the glucose supply is depleted, the body can raise the amount of fat it breaks down to use for energy. Excess amino acids, the essential components of protein, may be used to generate electricity. On the other hand, the body cannot use its own tissue as a food until you go weeks without feeding.

What about breaking the fast? What's the right way to do it?

Breaking the fast is one of the most difficult aspects of this lifestyle, and it's definitely the real litmus test on if you'll be able to stick with it long-term. For a variety of causes, it is essential to interrupt the fast in moderation. First and foremost, do not overload your system with too much at once since this will cause stress on your body and weaken your stomach and intestines if done too frequently. Furthermore, if you encourage yourself to binge while your determination is at its lowest, you are much more likely to binge and undo all of the diligent work you have already put in by Fasting.

Planning accordingly is the only approach to avoid this from happening. When you're waiting for the fast to stop, prepare the meal and make sure the portions are well specified.

Chapter 2: The Importance of Intermittent Fasting for Women over 50

Intermittent Fasting, in general, is beneficial for all age groups and genders, regardless of what individuals make out of it. But because this book is especially meant for aging women to help them discover their reroute to youth and secret to longevity, read this chapter to find out how you can do it.

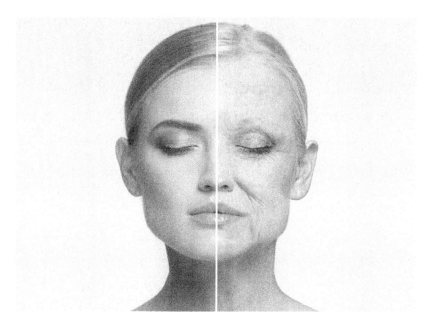

2.1 Understanding Autophagy – The 5 stages of Intermittent Fasting

Autophagy is the process of eating one's own body. Fasting has a lengthy and complicated series of effects on the body. Still, one of the most noticeable is the activation of a mechanism called autophagy, which simply means "self-eating." Autophagy is an entirely normal phenomenon that disintegrates and consumes dying, sick, or faded cells.

Consider the body to be similar to a vehicle. When everything is brand fresh, everything is vibrant and sparkling, and it functions properly. However, with time, pieces wear out, and some begin to rust. If you keep on driving it at fast speeds all the time, it would finally break down. Take the vehicle to a dealership so that technicians can remove and repair worn-out pieces and spruce it up and keep it running for as long as it takes. It is self-evident that you cannot fix the vehicle and push it hard simultaneously time. The same can be said for us. We need time away from relentless feeding, much like we need sleep, toggle on the repair genes that hold us in good health. Our bodies will only continue this repair phase when we are not consuming or consuming food with calories in it.

While Belgian biochemist Christian de Duve introduced the word "autophagy" in 1963, our knowledge of the phenomenon has advanced dramatically in this century, with Japanese biologist Yoshinori Ohsumi winning the Nobel Prize in 2016 for his observations and studies on the processes that underlie autophagy. That being said, as investigators are careful to point out, the science is still young, and much about autophagy stays unclear. Autophagy is "a method of cellular housekeeping" that is critical for "cellular quality control" and helps cells to properly "respond to stress," according to a few recent reports.

And is autophagy triggered by Fasting? It seems to, notwithstanding the fact that the majority of research on fasting-induced autophagy has been conducted in rodents. Clean eating and calorie limitation have long been linked to a slower aging process and a greater lifetime, but their precise function in autophagy activation is still unknown. "The literature largely [implies] that autophagy is caused in a large range of organs and tissues in reaction to caloric restriction," according to a 2018 study. Autophagy is a crucial step in cellular and molecular revitalization since it eliminates defective cellular elements, such as misfolded proteins. When the cells can't or won't activate autophagy, terrible things happen, like neurodegenerative disorders, which seem to be linked to decreased autophagy as people age. Fasting stimulates the AMPK signaling cascade and reduces motor function, causing autophagy to be activated. This is just when you've depleted your glucose reserves, and your blood sugar has dropped significantly. Autophagy improves in mice starved after 24 hours, and this phenomenon is amplified in liver and brain cells after 48 hours. Autophagy has been observed in human macrophages as early as 24 hours after fasting. Workout combined with calorie restriction through Fasting will boost autophagy in a variety of body glands.

Your growth hormone output is up to 5 times higher than when you began your fast after 48 hours lacking calories or very little calories, carbohydrates, or other nutrition. One explanation for this is that ketone particles formed during Fasting stimulate growth hormone release, which is beneficial to the brain. Ghrelin, the appetite hormone, also stimulates the development of growth hormone. Growth hormone aids in the preservation of lean body mass and the reduction of fat tissue deposition, especially as we get older. It can also contribute to human survival and encourage tissue repair and coronary protection.

2.2 How Intermittent Fasting Can Lead to A Longer Life?

There are several various diet programs from which to select. Some will assist you in limiting your carb consumption when focusing on healthy fats and proteins. Some people recommend limiting fat consumption and focusing on decent, nutritious carbohydrates.

With too many options on the market and at least a couple of them being viable weight-loss solutions, you might be wondering why you should choose intermittent Fasting. In this part, you'll learn about the different benefits of intermittent Fasting and how it can improve your well-being. It makes things easier. Although this isn't technically a health bonus like the rest, it's always worth mentioning. Intermittent Fasting has been shown to be beneficial to many individuals. They discover that as long as they remain within the hours required to feed, they don't have to worry about the calories they consume. They will go a couple of days a week without needing to prepare a meal. On the whole, this diet plan will help you live a better life.

You will reduce tension in your life by cutting out any of the things you need to do throughout the day and focusing on something else. We're both aware that too much work may be harmful to our wellbeing and wellbeing. It is much better to be a thveberion of yourself because you can reduce depression. It is beneficial to the heart. Heart disease is one of the leading causes of death worldwide. Any of these adverse outcomes, such as blood sugar levels, inflammation receptors, blood triglyceride levels, cholesterol, and heart rate, maybe helped by intermittent Fasting. The only problem is that several experiments on extended Fasting have been conducted on primates. More research into the effects of intermittent Fasting on human heart health is required. It can aid in the treatment of cancer. Per year, a large number of individuals are diagnosed with cancer. The unchecked development of cells is a defining feature of this horrific disease. Fasting has been found to have many health advantages, including improved appetite and a lower incidence of cancer. According to some human research, cancer patients who abstained were able to decrease any of the side effects of chemotherapy.

It is beneficial to the brain. What is beneficial to the body is often helpful to the brain. Intermittent Fasting has been seen to enhance metabolic features that are believed to aid in brain development. This may involve insulin tolerance, blood sugar control, inflammatory reduction, and cellular oxidative diminution. Intermittent Fasting has been seen in many experiments on rats to further develop fresh nerve cells, which increases the brain's work. Fasting will also aid in the rise of brain-derived neurotrophic factor levels. When the brain is lacking in this region, it may lead to depression and many other problems. It aids in cellular repair. When we're on a fast, our bodies' cells will start a waste-removal process known as autophagy. Such proteins that can no longer be utilized are broken down and metabolized by the cells. Autophagy could aid defend the body against diseases like Alzheimer's and cancer if it is enhanced. One of the most prevalent neurodegenerative disorders is Alzheimer's disease. Since there is no treatment for Alzheimer's disease, the safest action plan is to avoid it. Intermittent Fasting could prolong the progression of Alzheimer's disease, or at the very least, minimize its seriousness, according to a rat report. According to some case studies, a dietary change that involved some regular, or at least periodic, short-term fasts helped 9 out of 10 Alzheimer's patients relieve their symptoms. Fasting like this has also been shown in animal research to better guard against other neurodegenerative disorders like Huntington's and Parkinson's. While the majority of these experiments were conducted on primates, the findings seem to be positive. Intermittent Fasting is a fad, and research on how it benefits the body is only in its early stages. It would require time to research all of the advantages of intermittent Fasting. Intermittent Fasting can help you live a longer life. The fact that intermittent Fasting will help you live longer is one of the fascinating aspects of it. Several experiments on rats have shown that intermittent Fasting will help them live longer, close to what occurs when you go on a tight calorie-restricted diet. The results were dramatic in each of the experiments. When rats fasted every other day in one of the studies, they lived 83 percent longer than rats who did not fast. While it has been difficult to show an improvement in longevity because skipping breakfast has yet to be tested on people over a long enough period, it is nevertheless a common concept among those who want to delay aging. It's no surprise that people assume that intermittent Fasting can help them live longer and healthier lives, given the proven metabolic advantages of this lifestyle. If you see, there are many advantages of following an intermittent fasting diet. We have mentioned a handful, but there has been much research on the impact of this diet and why it could be beneficial to you. Intermittent Fasting will help you live

longer, lose weight and get more stamina if you're trying to boost your brain function, live longer, or lose weight.

Chapter 3: Exploring Different Diets During Intermittent Fasting

Now that you know what intermittent Fasting is and what role it can play for your health, it's time that you learn the various delicious recipes you can practice it with. Read this chapter to find out how you can deal with your desire to binge and different easy yet healthy diets you can try alongside Intermittent Fasting.

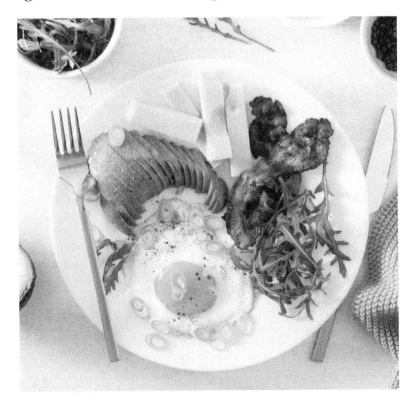

3.1 Identifying and Fighting Hunger Pangs

There's no need to be concerned with infrequent, short-term starvation. You will not die if your overall health is good. You won't crumble in a heap and need the cat's assistance. And if it has missed the ability due to years of eating, choosing, and snacking, your body is built to go without meals for lengthy periods. According to studies, contemporary people misinterpret a wide variety of hunger feelings. We feed when we're bored, thirsty, in the presence of food (when aren't we?), in the company of others, or literally when the clock tells us it's time to eat. Much of us feed because it makes us feel healthy. This is recognized as a 'hedonic appetite,' and while you can strive to fight it on a fast day, you should relax, knowing that you can succumb to pressure the next day if you like.

There's no reason to be concerned with it. Simply put, the human mind is capable of convincing us that we're starving in almost every circumstance: when confronted with emotions of scarcity, isolation, or unhappiness; when upset, sad, satisfied, or neutral; when subjected to ads, social imperatives, sensory gratification, incentive, habit, or the scent of black coffee or baking bread or bacon frying in a café down the lane. Recognize that these are mostly learned responses to external stimuli, most of which are intended to defraud you of your money. Suppose you're still digesting your last meal. In that case, it's extremely doubtful that you're hungry ('total transit period,' if you're interested in such stuff, can take up to two days, focusing on your sex, physiology, and what you've ingested).

Like a package of sharp blades, hunger pangs may be aggressive and unpleasant, but they are more flexible and manageable in reality than you would expect. You won't get hungry until you've been fasting for a long time. Furthermore, a pang will subside. Fasters claim that the sensation of hunger arrives in waves rather than as an ever-increasing wall of gnawing belly noise. It's a symphony with distinct gestures rather than a slow, terrifying crescendo. Consider a stomach rumble as a symbol of good health. Also, keep in mind that appetite does not grow over a 24-hour cycle, so don't get trapped by it at any given time. Wait a minute. You have complete control of your hunger feelings simply by directing your thoughts, riding the surge, and deciding to do something else — go for a stroll, call a buddy, drink tea, drive, shower, perform in the shower, call a friend from the shower, sing... Individuals often say that their appetite is reduced after a few weeks of observing Intermittent

Fasting. As it has been shown, one of the most important experiments on how obese subjects respond to Intermittent Fasting was conducted at the University of Chicago with volunteers using the more challenging Alternate-Day Modified Fasting process (ADMF). According to this report, 'Hunger scores were increased during the first week of Alternate-Day Modified Fasting. However, hunger scores decreased after two weeks of ADMF. They stayed poor for the remainder of the study, showing that subjects became habituated to the ADMF diet (i.e., experience very little hunger on a fast day) after approximately two weeks.' 'Enjoyment with the ADMF diet was poor during the first four weeks of the experiment, but steadily improved during the last four weeks of the trial,' according to the researchers.In brief, the researchers concluded that since appetite practically disappears and diet fulfillment skyrockets in a short span of time, obese participants are likely to stick to the diet over extended periods? Remember, this study was conducted with participants who fasted every single day, something we all attempted and found difficult. Partial Fasting two days a week, as recommended by the fast diet schedule, is much easier. But don't lose heart. Refrain, control, delay, and distract yourself on a fast day. You've reassigned your brain, and starvation is no longer an option.

3.2 Consumable and Non-Consumable Foods During Intermittent Fasting

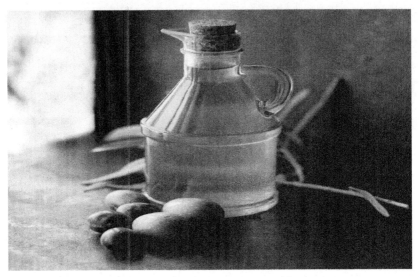

We've always heard the adage, "You are what you feed." For the most part, this means "avoid fast food." However, this familiar phrase represents a hidden reality. The diet you consume will affect how you act and look and whether you sleep soundly at night, whether you remain slim or respond immediately, and whether you have a pear-shaped or apple-shaped body. The amount of food you consume decides if your brain gets its energy from glucose or ketone bodies, and the amount and quality of food you eat will influence the odds of becoming pregnant if you're a woman. It's vital to consume foods you like, but it's also critical to avoid or limit foods that will shorten your life, make you sicker, and maximize your absorption of food that will improve your life healthier and easier.

Many additives are chemicals that cause extraordinary alterations, and shifts in their quantities and concentrations will modify the activity of our tissues and organs. Proteins, carbohydrates, fats, and micronutrients are also important components of a healthy diet. The food we consume contains three main ingredients, which we refer to as macronutrients.

Proteins are made up of twenty amino acids, the sequence of which specifies their role. A 3-ounce steak, for example, includes around 25 grams of protein. Actin, which is involved in muscle contraction and many other cellular processes, is one of the most prevalent proteins in meat. Meat is broken down into protein and then amino acids by the digestive system until it is consumed. These organic molecules are produced in two stages: first in the liver, then in the intestine. Simple amino acids or chains of several amino acids are ingested into the bloodstream. Amino acids are eventually spread to various cell types in the body, where they are used to produce new proteins, such as human muscle actin.

Carbohydrates may be present in most things, including in their basic form (such as the sugars in fruit juices, honey, sweets, or soft drinks) or in their complicated form (such as the long chains of glucose as well as other sugars found in vegetables and grains). Simple sugar will quickly reach the bloodstream, raising blood glucose levels, and prompt the pancreas to release insulin quickly. Until being consumed by the body, excess calories must be isolated from other food ingredients and decomposed into basic sugars.

There are a few different ways to evaluate a food's nutritional value regarding carbohydrates and their consistency. The words "glycemic index" and "glycemic load" are presumably familiar to you. The glycemic index of a product applies to how it affects blood glucose levels. Orange juice has a glycemic load of about 50, white bread has a glycemic index of 95, and a pure glucose beverage has a glycemic index of 100. The glycemic index, on the other hand, suggests that you consume a normal amount of carbohydrates. The glycemic load is a more accurate calculation since it shows both the properties and quantities of a given carbohydrate. Whole-wheat bread, for example, has a strong glycemic index but a low glycemic burden (a portion of whole bread). In comparison, sponge cake has a low glycemic index but a higher glycemic load. The glycemic load, which considers both the content and abundance of sugars in a meal, should be your primary concern.

In us and other mammalian and smaller animals, fats are the primary source of accumulated energy. Enhanced fat molecules also perform other important roles in the body's cells, along with a central function in the formation of the membrane that divides all cell material from the bloodstream and the production of hormones, especially steroids. Triglycerides, which are made up of three chains of carbon and hydrogen molecules (fatty acids) linked together by a glycerol molecule, are the most common type of fat consumed.

During absorption, bile salts produced from the gallbladder and lipase enzymes released from the pancreas and other organs break them down in the intestine so they can be ingested into the blood. Saturated fatty acids (those with the maximum amount of hydrogen atoms bound to every carbon) and unsaturated fats (those with less than the highest number of hydrogen atoms bound to each carbon) are the two types of fats. Monounsaturated fats (including the oleic acid used in olive oil) and polyunsaturated fats are two types of unsaturated fats (such as those found in salmon and corn oil). The polyunsaturated fats omega-3 and omega-6 are referred to as "necessary fatty acids" since they cannot be produced by the human body but are needed for proper cell and organ function.

Micronutrients are an essential component of the diet in comparison to the three main macronutrients. Like vitamins and minerals, Micronutrients make up a large portion of the $37 billion supplement market in the United States. Dr. Bruce Ames, a diet researcher, and others have shown that between 50 and 90 percent of US adults are deficient in vitamin D, E, magnesium, vitamin A, calcium, potassium, or vitamin K. Around the same period, several new studies have shown that nutritional supplements providing excessive vitamins and minerals are unsuccessful in avoiding major diseases and extending life expectancy.

One potential exception: a massive, randomized, regulated study found that people who took regular multivitamins had a slight decrease in leukemia and cataracts.

While high-dose vitamin and mineral supplements do not protect against aging or cancer, we know that they are important for many bodily functions. Vitamin D, zinc, and iron, for example, are important for proper immune function. Calcium and vitamin D are essential for healthy immune function. Calcium and vitamin D are important for skeletal muscle mass to remain normal.

And if a diet high in fruits, seafood, nuts, and whole grains is the best way to get the necessary nutrients, it may be low in vitamin D and, in the case of vegans and the elderly, vitamin B12. Most individuals who eat what is considered a high-nourishment lifestyle have identical deficits all around the planet. Since large doses of such vitamins have been shown in certain experiments to be harmful, the ideal prescription, according to both supporters and critics of supplement usage, is to take a multivitamin every 2 to 3 days that includes at least vitamin D, E, magnesium, vitamin A, calcium, potassium, or vitamin K.

It's important to replenish after you've gotten rid of the trash. It's just as bad to have no stuff in the fridge as it is to have a bunch of fast food. You would eventually eat. Takeout or a quick stop at the gas station for treats. Here are ten must-haves, all of which will come in handy while preparing the meals at the journal's back.

- A big bottle of extra virgin olive oil Doesn't be shy about it. When frying, use olive oil or organic rapeseed oil.

Also, grab a bottle of extra-virgin olive oil for greens.

- Plenty of veggies, including spinach, broccoli, cabbage, onions, cherry tomatoes, aborigines, carrots, cucumbers, and corvettes. If you just need something, chop up some broccoli, celery, or cucumber ahead of time to snack on. Place them near the top of the refrigerator, where they will be visible when you open the lid.

- Dairy goods with high-fat content also including full-fat or unsweetened yogurt, cheese, and cream. Real fats will hold you satisfied for better. A little piece of cheese with just some pear slices is the go-to lunch.

- Fizzy water and black tea are among the top ten beverages. Soda water will make you feel full without introducing calories per gram. To add flavor, add a slice of lemon, orange, or grapefruit. Herbal teas are yet another good substitute for sugary beverages. In most supermarkets, you'll notice a wide variety of flavors. Herbal tea can be kept cool in the refrigerator.

- Nuts and seeds that haven't been salted or sweetened. Almonds, cashews, Brazil nuts, hazelnuts, dried apricots, pine nuts, chia and walnuts are also good choices. To improve the flavor, roast them and store them in a pot. Nuts are high in fiber, which helps to fuel the microbiota, and they're also a good source of natural fat. But only eat a tiny handful at a time.

- If you're craving something nice, fruit is a perfect substitute for cakes and biscuits. But, restrict yourself to two bits per day and enjoy it during a meal instead of as a snack since it prevents ketosis (fat burning). Fruits with less sugar, such as grapes, strawberries, and pears, are a good option.

- Real grains like wild and brown rice, quinoa, and pearl barley. These may be substituted for white rice and pasta in small quantities in your meals. Try to get rid of as much bread as possible. While it is difficult, 'going chocolate' is impossible to decrease the amount of sugar consumed. If you want, have a slice of seeded cashew butter or dark rye bread.

- There are eggs. You should have eggs on hand at all times and eat them for breakfast most times of the week. They're high in protein which can leave you feeling satisfied for more time.

- Lentils and beans Legumes are high in dietary fiber and nutrients, whether they are dried, canned, or precooked in packages. They're normally better served with a drizzle of olive oil. Add a few to stews, salads, or baked goods. They're high in fiber, which is important for good microbiota.

- Fish with a lot of oil. Besides breakfast, grilled salmon fits well with eggs, and canned tuna makes a perfect snack or lunchtime choice. Smoked haddock is a flavorful and easy-to-prepare product. You can consume oily fish only twice every seven days.

3.3 The Keto Diet

The physiological condition of ketosis, the burning of ketones, a.k.a. ketone bodies, or the nutritional macronutrient structure (ultra-low-carb, moderate-protein, high-fat) that facilitates the acquisition of this fragile metabolic state are all referred to as "keto." Ketones are a caloric energy supply in the body and are utilized in the same way that glucose is for the brain, heart, and muscles (sugar). They are formed in the liver as a by-product of fat synthesis when insulin, blood sugar, and liver glycogen levels are extremely low due to dietary carbohydrate restriction. Most people never get close to this condition, and they never get to see the almost mystical effects of this organic super fuel. Ketones and fat (since these two caloric energy sources are both burned together) tend to reduce inflammation and oxidative harm caused by the western grain-based high-

carbohydrate diet. Keto understanding stems from the mainstream primal/paleo/low-carb dietary trend of the last decade. Still, it is more precise in terms of necessary dietary macronutrient levels, and it may be much more beneficial for weight reduction, disease prevention, and maximum neurological and athletic capacity than a traditional low-carb diet.

The advantages of extended Fasting and following a ketogenic diet should be obvious by now. The relation between the two, however, might have escaped your notice. When you're in ketosis, the body uses the same method of breaking down fatty acids to create ketones for food as it does when you're fasting. What does it imply to mix the two, and why should both lifestyles and eating habits be combined?

When consuming a conventional carb-centric diet, fasting for one or two days has a significant impact. Your body automatically turns to burn fat as fuel after the initial process of burning glucose (carbohydrates) for energy.

Imagine the consequences of mixing prolonged fasting with keto if it takes the body twenty-four to forty-eight hours to turn to consume fat for food. When the body is in a steady state of ketosis, it is still consuming fat for energy. This suggests that the more time you spend Fasting; the more calories you'll lose.

Intermittent Fasting mixed with keto boosts the effectiveness of Fasting's weight-loss results, resulting in greater weight loss than conventional diets. The longer period between your last and first meals of the day ensures your body has more fat-burning potential.

Ketosis is used in bodybuilding since it is a natural way to lose weight without sacrificing muscle mass. Weight reduction is beneficial only when it is at a stable level, and we all need body mass to maintain our wellbeing.

Switching to a ketogenic diet is a major lifestyle change. As a result, it's better to start slowly with the intermittent fasting portion of this method. Before integrating intermittent Fasting into your eating regimen, or in this situation, your prolonged duration of not eating, give your body time to adjust to a different way of eating; get used to burning fat for food, and cope with any potential side effects (remember, keto flu is a possibility). The 4-Week Plan would not incorporate intermittent Fasting until Week 2 of the program.

You should keep track of your eating hours throughout the phase-in process. Your last meal of the day should be no later than 6 p.m., even though you aren't using the intermittent fasting part of the schedule. This can help you get used to Fasting and stop snacking. Keto has the benefit of teaching your body—and, let's be honest, your brain—to feed only when you're hungry.

Cravings fade as time passes.

Cravings are frequently confused with hunger, but hunger is a natural call to replenish our energy stores, while cravings are a learned activity. It's up to you if you plan to incorporate your intermittent fasting period. If you want to enter the pool with your head first or with your toes first? Knowing this for yourself will assist you in deciding which routine is best for you.

Until you start, be aware of the following:

In every case, looking at the larger picture is important for long-term results. This is particularly true when making significant dietary and lifestyle adjustments. All you believed you learned about diet, when to eat, and what to eat goes out the window with intermittent keto.

Before getting started, familiarize yourself with what to anticipate, how to tackle future problems, and how to reorganize your life in a manner that allows you to accomplish your goals.

Define the objectives.

Why did you want to go on an irregular keto diet? Is it for the sake of your health? Is it possible to lose weight? Are you just looking to sleep stronger and have more energy? Is this a one-time cleanse, or are you looking to make long-term lifestyle changes? How do you want to monitor your macronutrient intake? Are you going to screen for ketones to make sure you're in ketosis? Can you eat a vegetarian or vegan diet?

All of these are crucial questions to think about before you start so you can remain concentrated on your target. Intermittent Fasting has been shown in studies to have significant long-term health effects. The jury is also out on the advantages and dangers of following a ketogenic diet indefinitely. The rigidity of the schedule often determines how long people stick to it.

When it comes to keto, the way you diet is still important to remember because you should be aware of how much of a transition or obstacle this would be. In terms of macronutrients, keto is a fat-focused diet, but protein plays a significant part. During ketosis, too little protein may lead to muscle weakness. On the other hand, you might lose your ketosis if you overeat. It's a compromise because although keto isn't a high-protein diet, meat is often seen as the default protein since plant-based protein substitutes, such as beans and tofu, are usually too high in carbohydrates relative to their fiber and protein ratios (which is made from soybeans). This isn't to say that staying vegetarian on keto is difficult, particularly if you're an ovo-lacto vegetarian (okay with eating eggs and dairy). Eggs, nuts and beans, and cheese are examples of non-meat protein options that aren't legumes.

3.4 The Plant Diet

You've always learned that processed foods are terrible for you before. "Prevent preservatives; ban packaged goods," they say, but no one tells you why you should prevent them or why they are unhealthy. So, let's break things down so you can see that you can stay away from these bad guys.

They have a lot of addictive qualities. We have a clear predisposition to become hooked to such things as humans, but it is not solely our responsibility. Almost all of the toxic foods we consume from time to time stimulate the dopamine neurotransmitter throughout our brain. This temporarily helps the brain feel "nicer," but just for a brief time. This leads to an obsession, which is why someone would still catch themselves reaching for that snickers bar, even though they shouldn't need one. All of this would be avoided by suppressing the stimuli entirely.

Sugar and high fructose corn syrup are abundant. Sugars and high fructose corn syrup, which have almost no health benefit, are abundant in processed and animal-based foods. More and more experiments show what many people already knew: genetically engineered diets exacerbate intestinal inflammation, which makes it difficult for the body to consume vital nutrients. The consequences of your body struggling to consume vital nutrients, which range from muscle weakness to brain fog to weight gain, cannot be overstated. There are a lot of processed sugars in them. Refined carbohydrates are abundant in processed foods and animal-based items. Carbohydrates are used by your body to supply energy for normal body functions. On the other hand, synthesizing carbs removes the essential nutrients, much as refining whole grains removes the whole grain portion. After refining, you're left with what's known as "empty" carbohydrates. Through peaking, your blood sugar and insulin levels will have a detrimental effect on your digestion.

They include ingredients that allow the body to feel a surge of pleasure. This ensures that they can include substances such as monosodium glutamate (MSG), high fructose corn syrup elements, and some dyes that have addictive properties. They activate the body to get a reward. MSG, for example, is used in several pre-packaged pastries. This activates your taste buds, allowing you to appreciate the flavor. The way your subconscious interacts with your taste buds makes it psychological. This reward-based system causes the body to crave even more of it, placing you at risk of calorie excess.

They're full of fake additives. Artificial ingredients are treated as alien objects by the body when you consume them. They basically transform into intruders. The human body doesn't recognize sucralose and other chemical sweeteners. As a result, the body does what it does well: it does what it does best. It activates an immune reaction, lowering the tolerance and rendering you more susceptible to disease. Your body's attention and energies may otherwise be drawn away from defending your immune system.

What about protein derived from animals?

Plant proteins are sometimes referred to as "poor quality" since they have less basic amino acids than animal proteins. Many people are unaware that consuming so many basic amino acids may be harmful to your body. So, let's have a look at how it works.

Animal protein is deficient in fiber. Many citizens wind up dispersing the plant protein they do have in their search for more animal protein. Animal protein, unlike plant protein, is sometimes deficient in fiber, vitamins, and micronutrients. Fiber loss is very widespread in many cultures and societies around the world. As per the Institute of Medicine, the typical adult in the United States eats just around 15 grams of fiber a day, compared to the recommended 38 grams. Dietary fiber deficiency has been linked to an elevated incidence of colon and breast cancers, as well as Crohn's disease, cardiac disease, and constipation.

IGF-1 levels rise as animal protein is consumed. Insulin-like growth factor-1 (IGF-1) is a hormone. It promotes cell division and expansion, which can seem positive, but it also promotes cancer cell development. IGF-1 levels in the blood are therefore linked to an elevated risk of disease, malignancy, and proliferation. Phosphorus levels rise as animal protein is consumed. This is because the phosphorus content of animal protein is high. Our bodies regulate elevated phosphorus levels by secreting a hormone known as fibroblast growth factor 23. (FGF23). According to a 2013 report named "Circulating Fibroblast Growth Factor 23 Is Associated with Angiographic Severity and Extent of Coronary Artery Disease," this hormone is toxic to our blood vessels. FGF23 has also been linked to irregular cardiac muscle enlargement, which contributes to heart disease and, in rare circumstances, death.

Given the above concerns, animal protein's "good quality" component could be better characterized as "high risk." Except for caffeine, which causes addiction once you are taking it fully, refined foods may be stopped immediately. Perhaps the most important thing you'll miss is not needing to cook a single meal from scratch.

Chapter 4: Methods of Intermittent Fasting

If you'd like to burn calories, shed pounds, and stay in better condition, intermittent Fasting is a perfect choice. This lifestyle is about more than just the things you consume. It's more about whether you consume these things so that you can stay balanced and have your body perform the heavy lifting for you.

The most difficult aspect of this lifestyle is teaching yourself not to feed constantly. We've been told that we can consume four to six meals a day (which is good if they're small), but this isn't true for most people. You will achieve the results you like without needing to try as much if you use extended Fasting. There are hence, various methods of IF which you can try and decide to opt for. This chapter has briefly discussed the most common yet popular ones for you.

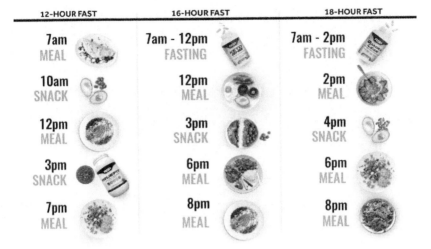

12-HOUR FAST	16-HOUR FAST	18-HOUR FAST
7am MEAL	**7am - 12pm** FASTING	**7am - 2pm** FASTING
10am SNACK	**12pm** MEAL	**2pm** MEAL
12pm MEAL	**3pm** SNACK	**4pm** SNACK
3pm SNACK	**6pm** MEAL	**6pm** MEAL
7pm MEAL	**8pm** MEAL	**8pm** MEAL

4.1 The 5:2 Fast

The 5:2 method of intermittent Fasting is among the most common and simplest method for beginners to try. As the ratio suggests, 5 days are your normal feeding days, whereas 2 days of the week are reserved for Fasting. The only difficult part is that you have to restrict your calorie take on those 2 days by 70 to 80%.

The 5:2 diet is easy to try nonetheless and has several benefits to offer. The findings of a long-term analysis testing the impact of the 5:2 on people with higher blood sugar levels were released in July 2018 by an Australian community located at the Sansom Institute of Health Research.

To give you an indication of how long these studies take,

the Australians began preparing this one in 2014, finished it by the end of 2017, and released the findings in July 2018. For the report, 137 overweight or obese people with high blood sugar levels were randomly assigned for a year on either the 5:2 solution or a traditional weight loss diet. Both groups were provided detailed booklets on their respective diets, along with sample meals, and sent away to get on with it after being carefully weighed and calculated. This research is unique because the participants were not offered specific diets or meal supplements, nor were they given a lot of expert guidance, as is usual in diet studies. They simply received counseling and were given monthly visits with a professional dietician during the first six months.

The aim was to simulate real-world reality rather than anything that could only be achieved with a lot of money and expert support. So, what went wrong? Over the first ninety of the research, all classes were excellent at keeping to their diets, with 97 percent of 5:2 individuals and 90 percent of those on a normal diet remaining on board. However, about a third of the participants had avoided following their assigned diet by completing the year, whether because they had met their targets or because they were bored of dieting. The regular dieters have a higher dropout rate than the 5:2 dieters. Indeed, the 5:2 individuals discovered that if they had to abandon the diet for some cause, it was simple to resume – while those on the regular diet appeared to give up for betterment.

Whereas, as far as weight loss is concerned, the individuals who were assigned to the 5:2 diet lost a total of 7.1 kg and held it off. That's 2.1 kg heavier than the average dieter. They have shed more weight, and their blood glucose levels improved significantly. Few people performed better than others. The top 20% of the 5:2 individuals lost and held off an average of 12.5 kilograms, which was 4 kilograms higher than the top 20% of the normal dieting community. The 5:2 diet is healthy and successful in individuals with type 2 diabetes, according to the experts, as long as it is closely controlled.

Dr. Michelle Harvie and Professor Tony Howell of Manchester University released the findings of a report on the impact of two days of calorie restriction on 115 middle-aged women shortly after The fast Diet was published in 2013. Three classes of women were formed. One party was told to adhere to a 1500-calorie Mediterranean diet, and the other (dubbed "two-day dieters") was told to consume a 650-calorie, low-carbohydrate Mediterranean diet five days a week and a

650-calorie, low-carbohydrate variant the other two days. A third party was required to avoid carbs for two days per week but was not limited in any other way.

After 90 days, the two-day dieters had lost a total of 6 kg, almost twice as much as the normal dieters, and had lost significantly more belly fat. In addition, the insulin tolerance of the two-day dieters improved much more than that of the normal dieters. Those who followed the two-day plan for more than three months dropped an average of 6 pounds, with some losing more than 14 pounds. So, just another reassuring analysis for those considering a 5:2 diet. Dr. Harvie recently requested 23 overweight, premenopausal women at elevated cancer incidence to restrict their calorie intake during one menstrual period on two days a week. They wanted to provide breast biopsies in addition to the normal examinations. Over the span of a month, the participants not only shed a total of 3 kg, the majority of which was body fat, but they also had substantial increases in the activity of genes linked to breast cancer in the majority of them.

Charles Dickens once wrote, "Get a spirit that never hardens." It's good guidance, even though he didn't mean it medically.

Following dementia, heart disease is the second leading cause of death in the United Kingdom. And if you endure a heart attack, that will have long-term consequences. Despite its status as a common sign of passion, the heart is simply an excellent pump. It's the size of a palm and pumps five liters of blood into your body's 96,500 kilometers of blood vessels 70 times per minute. That's 100,000 times a day, and if you hold it in decent condition, it can continue to do so for the next three billion years. The problem is that many of us have aging organs quicker than we should, which might explain why they are often the first component of the human machine to fail.

So, how can you hold your heart in good shape?

You will reduce the chances of developing a heart attack or stroke by following a good diet (look up for the keto or plant based diet in the previous chapter), staying healthy and lowering tension. The 5:2 diet will also help you reduce weight and lower your blood sugar levels, which can boost your heart health. In a recent survey, 13 27 overweight men and women were randomly assigned to one of two diets: a 5:2 diet or a normal diet, with the aim of losing 5% of their body weight. Those on the 5:2 diet took 59 days to complete the task, while those on the regular diet took 73 days. Those who fasted saw a much greater drop in blood pressure (down 9 percent relative to 3 percent). The researchers discovered that while the dieters were given a fatty meal, the individuals who fasted were able to remove the fat from their bloodstream much more quickly. As a consequence, the 5:2 ratio was once again very promising.

4.2 The 8:16 Fast

IF may be practiced in a variety of ways. They do share one thing in common: they all have an eating cycle and an abstinence period.

The fasting interval differs in duration depending on the process used. You either consume nothing or drink zero-calorie drinks during this period. The feeding interval ranges in duration depending on the process. You can eat anything you want during this period, as long as you don't overeat. It's best if you diet regularly rather than as if you're making up for the time you went without calories. Such diets, such as The Warrior Diet, enable you to consume those items in a specific sequence.

Before we get into the 16:8 diet, it's necessary to note that intermittent fasting isn't for everybody. For example, intermittent fasting ought not to be attempted by the following people:

- Individuals under the age of 18

- Diabetics (both type 1 and type 2) who have not seen a doctor

- People with elevated cortisol levels

- Expecting and breastfeeding moms

- Individuals with disordered eating; people with insufficient body fat

Note: See a doctor or other qualified practitioner before starting any diet, physical fitness regimen, or changing your daily behaviors.

Let's have a closer look at the 16:8 approach in particular. This method is split into two phases, a 16-hour fasting cycle and a particular 8-hour eating period, as the title suggests. It's crucial that you stick to a consistent feeding schedule. This ensures you can't expect to eat from 8 a.m. to 4 p.m. today and then snack from 8 p.m. to 4 a.m. tomorrow. It is for the purpose of having an easy-to-follow routine that your body will respond to. Recollect how ghrelin, the appetite hormone, is produced in response to your eating habits? Modifying your pattern regularly could make you hungry all of the time and mess with your receptors.

One of the more popular strategies for intermittent fasting is to eat as little as possible. It necessitates fasting for 14 to 16 hours a day and eating for the rest of the time. You will easily get two or three meals in during this

feeding time. This is more apt to work with your regular diet routine, but it also restricts you enough that you don't snack every day. This approach is far simpler than you may believe. It's as simple as not consuming some snacks after dinner and then missing, or at the very least eating a late meal. So, if you take your last meal at 8 p.m. and don't eat it else before noon the very next day, you've now fasted for 16 hours. What you have to do now is be cautious with late-night snacks. If you consume them, you'll have to skip breakfast the next day. This practice is claimed to be more economical and easy to follow since it does not involve going without food over extended periods of time. Thus, it will comfortably blend into most people's daily lives. The average human, for example, sleeps for eight hours. When alive, you need to diet for another 8 hours, making the fasting time seem quicker.

If the last meal was at 10 p.m., you would fast before 2 p.m. the next day, most of which you will be sleeping and the other of which you will be busy with work - you will not realize the hour.

This approach is common since you can still have supper with friends or family until your eating window shuts.

Important Note: According to some studies, feeding late at night causes higher blood sugar spikes than feeding during the day, affecting sleep quality and encouraging nighttime processing.

Some people struggle with this when they are starving first thing in the morning and believe they must have breakfast. Breakfast will easily be rescheduled for afterward in the day. For e.g., if you have breakfast at 10 a.m. instead of 8 a.m. and then finish eating by 6 p.m., you'll always be inside the 16-hour span. If you're a woman, you should probably choose this choice. Women usually benefit from shorter fasts, and they will want to try staying 14 to 15 hours between meals since it is more convenient for them. You are permitted to consume non-caloric drinks such as tea, coffee, caffeine, and other non-alcoholic beverages during the fast to help relieve food cravings. Additionally, during your feeding period, you can aim to adhere to healthy items. Eating a lot of fatty food during this period is not a smart idea.

When doing an intermittent fast, certain people choose to eat a low-carb diet because it deals with appetite and improves outcomes.

4.3 The 20:4 Fast or the Warrior Diet

Ori Hofmelker, a health and wellbeing blogger, created the Warrior Diet, an intermittent fasting regimen. The diet consists of a long cycle of fasting accompanied by a brief period of supper. After years of studying himself and his teammates in the Israeli Special Forces, Hofmelker established the Warrior Diet in 2001.

Fasting is not a novel idea. Fasting is said to have originated in ancient Greece, where philosopher Pythagoras extolled the benefits of fasting. Fasting was advocated by Hippocrates and other influential healers, such as the Renaissance doctor Paracelsus. Food prohibition is also an essential part of certain traditions. Throughout the year, Judaism recognizes several fasting days; Muslims diet during the holy month of Ramadan, and several Catholics fast for 40 days throughout Lent. As demonstrated by the Suffragette crackdowns and Mahatma Gandhi's starvation periods during the movement for Indian freedom, fasting has often been used as a means of political agitation. Owing to promising outcomes from various weight-loss trials, fasting, also recognized as extended fasting, has now become a common method in the fitness modern age.

Intermittent fasting is just as it looks like: a time of fasting preceded by food, with the duration of the fast varying based on which procedure you obey. The Warrior Diet involves fasting for 20 hours and only feasting for four hours. During this time, the feasting part allows you to consume 85–90% of your calories. For anyone with a standard 2,000-calorie weight-management diet, this would be up to 1,800 calories in one sitting, or up to 2,700 calories, resting with a healthy person who wants 3,000 kcal a day. The Warrior Diet requires people to fast for 20 hours throughout the day and night time, then overeat for four hours each night. This approach is founded on the assumption that our forefathers lived their days searching and collecting and feasted at night. Hofmelker recommends eating limited amounts of dairy, hard-boiled eggs, and raw fruit throughout the fasting period. Water, chocolate, and milk are also zero-calorie or low-calorie drinks. To guarantee that you receive sufficiently essential nutrients and vitamins, it's a smart idea to eat a few portions of fruit and vegetables during the day. During the 4-hour feeding time, there are no limits. Although you might theoretically order a pizza, it's better to eat balanced, nutritious foods like fruits, vegetables, and meat. Whole-grain foods, including sprouted wheat flour, quinoa, grain, bulgur,and granola, are all excellent choices for fueling up through your feeding window. Protein is recommended, and organic and full-fat dairy foods; Hofmelker enjoys butter, yogurt, and raw milk. Like in every diet, certain foods and drinks you can strive to limit, such as those rich in sugar and salt. The Warrior Diet isn't focused on medicine in the scientific sense; however, the 20:4 regimens are focused on Hofmelker's own experience and views on the techniques he used to keep healthy during his army duty.

What You Should Do?

You can eat very few calories over the 20-hour fasting cycle. When it's convenient for your eating window, you will basically consume as much as you like before the four hours are completed. You can choose your eating window depending on whatever timeline fits best for you, but many individuals prefer to eat in the evening. When it comes to feasting, Hofmelker recommends focusing on healthier fats and vast sections of protein, especially dairy protein sources, including cheese and yogurt. If you obey Hofmelker's advice and eat only unprocessed ingredients, you won't need to measure calories on the Warrior Diet. Timing is a crucial aspect of this method. According to the program, long cycles of abstinence and short hours of overeating contribute to optimum well-being, nutrition, and body structure.

4.4 The 24 Hour Fast or the OMAD Diet

Simply stated, the one meal a day (OMAD) lifestyle entails fasting for 23 hours a day and consuming whatever you like for one meal. The meal could be anything from a double cheeseburger and fries to a salad of greens, roasted vegetables, whole grains, beans, nuts, and seeds. The premise is that if you restrict your calorie intake during the day, you will eat a big meal (generally a one-hour window) and yet stay slim. Water and unflavored tea and coffee are permitted, but the dining room is locked for the day.

So is there a difference between the OMAD diet and intermittent fasting? A one-meal-a-day Diet is a form of time-restricted intermittent fasting in which dieters fast for 12 hours or more per day. It is, of course, 23 in this situation. Most people accomplish this by fasting overnight, avoiding sleep, then taking their first meal in the afternoon of the day, leaving them with only seven hours to fantasize about food before heading to bed. The one-meal-a-day Diet is so severe that it renders other forms of fasting seem mild. The 16:8 Diet, for instance, allows you to feed for eight hours (between 9 a.m. and 5 p.m.) and abstain for the remaining 16. Alternate day fasting, frequently referred to as the 5:2 Diet, involves restricting the calorie consumption for several days per week and consuming normal meals and treats on the other days.

When you only consume one meal a day, you're probably getting far fewer calories than you would usually. Diminished calorie consumption typically leads to weight loss; large-scale trials have shown that those who fasted and others who merely lowered calorie consumption lose the very same bit of load. When following the OMAD diet, it's possible to feel depleted, contributing to bingeing and slipping off the wagon. Weight cycling (also known as "yo-yo dieting") and improvements to appetite hormones and metabolism are common during lengthy stretches of restraint. Finally, you feel hungrier after attempting the one-meal-a-day Diet than you did before beginning this restrictive program. It's not realistic for all of us to avoid Diet completely for fixed amounts of time to create food decisions that contribute to improved health and weight loss.

Intermittent fasting is designed to allow the essential organs, proteolytic juices, and metabolic processes a "break" while also lowering oxidative stress. Fasting, according to practitioners, increases the efficiency of organ tissues, decreases inflammation, and decreases the likelihood of chronic illness. It's also linked to a reduction in insulin tolerance, which may mean a reduced chance of diabetes.

Even so, there is strong proof that any advantage is easily reversed if you crack the hard, allowing craving hormones to turn gears and making you feel much hungrier than you did before. One possible benefit of time-restricted fasting is that it can encourage you to go to bed early, which is an essential part of any weight-loss strategy. Weight loss, decreased incidence of chronic illness, and increased metabolic effects have also been attributed to getting eight hours of sleep a night.

Chapter 5: The Role Of Intermittent Fasting In Menopause

You will find that keeping your normal weight gets more complicated when you grow older. In reality, many people accumulate weight when they approach menopause. That being said, weight gain after menopause is not unavoidable. You will change your life by focusing on healthier food behaviors and maintaining an active life. These hormonal imbalances can lead to weight gain over your abdomen rather than your buttocks and thighs. However, hormone fluctuations alone do not often result in weight gain after menopause.

In certain cases, body weight is caused by aging, as well as dietary and hereditary causes.

Hence you must consider pursuing a more active lifestyle and healthier diet, so what's better than intermittent fasting.

Read this chapter to find out what intermittent fasting can do for your aging body during menopause.

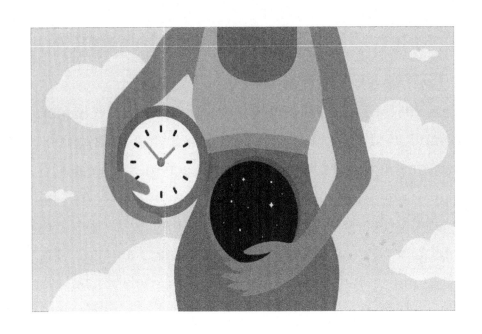

5.1 How Can Intermittent Fasting Aid in Menopause?

Periods, puberty, breastfeeding, and possibly postpartum depression. What a ride it is for most women. Then there's menopause, a hormone transformation period in women's lives that can be mentally, spiritually, and socially challenging. After generations of being committed to infants, husbands, and jobs, females in this process might be rediscovering themselves. Alternatively, they may be busier than ever, caring for elderly parents and college-aged children. (Who simply decides to stay.)

In either case, becoming older also prompts a need to reflect on one's fitness. Intermittent fasting has piqued the attention of certain women due to its connection to durability. Those around simply choose to lose weight in a simple manner. Although there isn't enough evidence to say if intermittent fasting is helpful to menopausal or postmenopausal people, we do know that limiting food is a stressor.

People concerned with restricting their food consumption to maintain a healthy weight have higher amounts of cortisol, a stress response, than women that aren't. Add in the sleep disturbances that come with menopause, and your "heat bucket" is quickly filling up. Lower estrogen levels also indicate a reduced body's ability to cope with stress. The bucket is filling up a lot faster than it used to be. And although certain stimuli are beneficial to our health, such as fitness, learning, and improvement, we will only become healthier if we allow ourselves to rebound from them. If you're a woman going through this hormonal process, just consider intermittent fasting if:

- Your anxiety level is not very accelerated.

- You're having a good night's sleep.

- Heart palpitations and mood fluctuations don't bother you.

- There are no food shortages in your body.

Until you get into the vegetation meat of this, get one thing straight:

1. Before making any significant lifestyle changes, it's still a good idea to consult with your respected medical professionals.

2. Although there is an increasing body of literature pointing to the health and cognitive advantages of Intermittent Fasting (IF), which we'll get to in a moment, we at Pause Well-Aging are "diet agnostic."

Rochelle Weitzner, our manager, and CEO, is a great supporter of the keto diet. However, we agree that coping with the all-too-common weight gain associated with menopause is a singular experience. What works wonders for one woman cannot lift the needle at all for another. So bide your time to do new things. Menopause isn't slipping away anytime soon.

Now, back to the subject at finger: Intermittent Fasting and its effectiveness for assisting us in losing menopause-related excess weight, especially those extra pounds that appear to cluster around our midsections. (It isn't your imagination that fastening a pair of trousers in your wardrobe has recently become significantly more complicated.) Connect the that perhaps the enzyme lipoprotein lipase has a substantial impact on where we accumulate fat in our bodies. Fat appears to cluster between our hips and buttocks when we're smaller. As we become older and closer to menopause, our hormone levels decrease, and fat tends to migrate to the belly. As a result, we now have pants-buttoning problems when we once had a natural waist. Surplus belly fat, described as a waist size of >35 inches for women, is terrible for us and has been related to a slew of medical conditions, including:

- Health attack/complications in the heart

- A stoke

- Diabetes type 2

- Hypertension and high blood cholesterol are two of the most common health problems.

- Breast and bowel cancer are two types of cancer.

Isn't it a great motivator to lose the 1.5 pounds we gain on average per year when we approach middle age? That's what we think. Although we can't limit weight reduction to a specific body region, losing pounds all over will eventually result in a leaner midsection. Intermittent fasting is a calorie-reduction technique that will help one lose weight and get rid of the dreaded "menopot."

In summary, Intermittent Fasting is the reduction of one's "food window" into a fixed amount of hours - or days, as the case may be, which we'll discuss further down. In other terms, rather than feeding as soon as you wake up and finishing with a pre-bed bowl of Haagen-Dazs at 11 p.m. (kindly don't do this), you schedule your meals from 10 a.m. to 6 p.m. You might wonder why someone would put themselves through all of this. Isn't it enough that we still have plenty on our tables without being hungry from fasting? So here's the thing about IF: after you've gotten used to it, you won't be hungry any longer. And if you find yourself in dire need of a snack, just respond to your body, get a nutritious snack, and move on about your day.

Fasting daily has a plethora of benefits for those experiencing menopause. IF has been attributed to a long list of health advantages, in addition to lowering the number of calories we eat - because no matter how you cut it, losing weight comes down to calories ingested versus calories spent - It improves "cardiovascular" fitness by controlling insulin levels and preventing pre-diabetes. It improves cognitive activity and "neuroplasticity," or the brain's capacity to create and reorganize neuronal associations, as well as lowering blood pressure, triglycerides, and cholesterol. In the end, if you're sick of not being able to fit into your pants, you may want to try Intermittent Fasting.

5.2 The Ideal IF Diet During Menopause

It's always been easy to eat just 500 calories a day if you deprive yourself. Consider certain low-calorie frozen meals, each with less than 300 calories. The servings are so small that they seem to be appetizers rather than main courses. And they're usually full of low-cost recipes you'd never prepare yourself. The positive thing is that you don't have to deprive yourself by restricting your calorie consumption to 500 calories. You can consume natural food and still be happy. Load up on protein, healthier fats, and fiber while avoiding calorie-dense basic carbohydrates like white sugar and flour. Protein can be obtained from any vegetable or animal products, and fiber can be obtained from fruits and vegetables.

Learning to cook teaches you about portion management and quality foods and allows you to consume real food. To keep under 500 calories for the day, simply change your food consumption accordingly.) They're easy to make, thanks to the Recipes in this chapter. You can get your evening meals and enjoy them too by consuming these protein-rich portions (that also keep you happy for a lot longer after you consume them) and incorporating balance in the form of salads, good fats, and fruits.

You should mix and match these dishes to your heart's content. And better, the majority of these recipes serve two individuals so that you can make plenty for two meals or exchange with a friend. To serve a large group, simply double or triple the recipes.

Cobb Salad with Chicken

Time to prepare: 15 minutes

· Time to cook: none

· Yield: 2 servings

- 5 cups Romaine lettuce, chopped
- 6 oz. fried, boneless, and skinless chicken breasts, diced (baked or grilled)
- 12 cup plum tomatoes, sliced
- 4 hard-boiled eggs, whites only, minced
- 1 cup unpeeled diced cucumber
- 1/2 cup cooked beets, diced
- 1/2 cup carrots, shredded

Directions:

1. On two dinner plates, arrange the broccoli.

2. Place a strip of chicken on top of the lettuce. Arrange the onions, eggs, cucumber, beets, and carrots in separate strips over the lettuce next to the bird.

3. In a medium mixing cup, whisk together all of the dressing components. Serve the salad with the sauce drizzled over it.

Grapefruit, Almonds, and Curried Coconut Dressing on Turkey Salad

Time to prepare: 5 minutes

· Time to cook: none

· Yield: 2 servings

Ingredients:

- 8 ounces cooked turkey breast meat, sliced into 1-inch pieces Ingredients

- 1 medium grapefruit, peeled, sliced into 1-inch pieces, separated into parts

- 1/4 cup slivered almonds 34 cup celery

- 1/4 cup coconut milk 2 teaspoons cilantro leaves, minced

- 2 tbsp. freshly squeezed lemon juice

- curry powder (1 teaspoon)

- 1/2 teaspoon garlic, minced

Directions:

1. To taste, season with fine sea salt and freshly ground pepper.

2. In a big mixing bowl, combine all of the ingredients and toss well to cover. To taste, season with salt and pepper.

Slow-Cooked Skinny Chili

Time to prepare: 30 minutes

· Time to cook: 5 hours

· Yield: 2 servings

Ingredients:

- 8 oz. ground beef (very lean)

- 1 cup water 1 cup diced tomatoes in juice from a can

- 1/4 cup celery, chopped 14 cup onions, chopped

- tablespoons chili ice (medium)

- 2 1/2 tablespoons garlic, ground

- a pinch (or more) of red pepper flakes

- a pinch of oregano, dried

- 12 teaspoon sea salt, perfect

- black pepper, freshly roasted

- 1 cup quarter-inch zucchini dice

- teaspoons scallion, diced

Directions:

1. Brown the ground beef in a big nonstick skillet over medium-high heat, often stirring to split up lumps. Combine all of the ingredients (except the zucchini) in a compact (3- to 4-quart) slow cooker with the browned beef.

2. Cook for 4 hours on low heat, covered. Heat for another hour after adding the zucchini and stirring well.

3. Season to taste with salt and pepper, and serve immediately with scallions on top.

Chapter 6: The Biological Benefits of Intermittent Fasting

Hormones and other significant chemicals in the body are often correlated with attitude, often play a significant part in the decision to lose weight. The release of these hormones from multiple glands is activated for many purposes. The pancreas, for example, releases insulin when blood sugar levels increase, which plays a role for diabetics and other severe disease sufferers. Read this chapter to find out what IF can do for your body's physiology.

6.1 Diabetes and Intermittent Fasting

Insulin is a fat-producing hormone. When we consume carbohydrate-rich foods, our blood sugar level levels increase, and the pancreas, an organ located far below ribs and around the left kidney, begins to produce insulin. While glucose is the primary energy source for our cells, the body dislikes getting large amounts of it flowing in the blood. Insulin is a chemical that regulates blood glucose levels, keeping them from being too high or too low. It usually does so with great accuracy. The issue arises when the pancreas is overworked.

Insulin is a glucose control system; it helps absorb glucose from the blood and then retains it in a safe form called glycogen in areas like the liver or muscles, ready to be utilized as and if required. Insulin is also a fat controller and is less well established. Lipolysis, or the secretion of accumulated body fat, is inhibited by it. Simultaneously, it causes fat cells to absorb and accumulate fat from the blood. Insulin is a fattening hormone. High levels promote fat accumulation, although low levels promote fat loss. The problem with consuming a ton of sugary, carbohydrate-rich snacks and beverages all of the time, like we continually do, is that the glucose rush necessitates the production of ever more insulin to cope with it. Your pancreas can cope past a certain point by actually pouring out greater and larger amounts of insulin, which results in a fatter deposition as well as an increased chance of cancer. Naturally, this cannot last indefinitely. Your cells will gradually revolt and become immune to the influence of insulin if you manage to generate greater amounts of it. It's similar to yelling at your kids; you may keep worsening the situation, but eventually, they'll quit listening. After your cells cease reacting to insulin, your blood sugar levels will remain permanently elevated, and you will join the 285 million people worldwide who have type 2 diabetes. It is a huge and exponentially expanding issue all over the planet. Numbers have almost tenfold increased in the last 20 years, and there is no evidence that this development is declining.

Diabetes is linked to a higher incidence of heart disease, stroke, impotence, blindness, and amputation of limbs due to inadequate circulation. It's also linked to aging and brain shrinkage. It's not a beautiful sight. Cutting down on carbs and replacing them with more vegetables and fat, which do not trigger such significant increases in blood glucose, is one way to avoid the downward diabetes slide. They still don't have too

In a 2005 survey, eight fit young men were required to fast every other day for two weeks, for a total of 20 hours. They were permitted to feed until 1 p.m. on fasting days and not feed again until 6 p.m. the following evening. They were even told that they needed to eat a lot the majority of the time to avoid losing weight.

The purpose of this experiment was to evaluate the so-called 'thrifty theory,' which states that since humans developed through a period of feast and famine, the safest way to eat is to eat like that. There were no improvements in the volunteers' weight or body fat distribution at the end of the two weeks, just what the researchers wanted. Their insulin sensitivity, on the other hand, has significantly improved. In other words, the same level of circulating insulin has a considerably stronger impact on the volunteers' capacity to retain glucose or decompose fat after only two weeks of Intermittent Fasting. 'By subjecting stable men to periods of feast and famine, we improved their metabolic state for the better,' the researchers wrote ecstatically. 'To our understanding, this is the first work in humans using Intermittent Fasting to achieve an improved insulin secretion on whole system glucose absorption and adipose tissue lipolysis,' they continued.

6.2 Cancer and Intermittent Fasting

Our bodies' cells replicate at a rapid rate, replacing dying, worn-out, or weakened tissue. This is great as long as cellular development is regulated, but a cell will mutate, expand uncontrollably, and eventually become cancerous. The presence of elevated amounts of a neuronal stimulus in the blood, such as IGF-I, is likely to raise the chances of this occurring.

Surgery, chemotherapy, and radiotherapy are the standard treatments for cancer that have gone rogue. Chemotherapy and radiotherapy are used to attempt to weaken the tumor, while surgery is used to try to extract it. Chemotherapy and radiotherapy have a significant drawback in that they are not selective; in addition to destroying tumor cells, they often destroy or harm healthy cells. They are particularly prone to harm quickly splitting cells like hair roots, which is why hair often falls out during treatment.

Valter Longo has demonstrated that when we are starved for even brief stretches of time, our bodies adapt by decelerating, heading into recovery and survival mode before food becomes plentiful again. Normal cells are the same way. Cancer cells, on the other hand, have their own set of laws. They are, perhaps by necessity, uncontrollable and would continue to increase selfishly regardless of the circumstances. This 'selfishness' opens up a window of chance. At least in principle, fasting right before treatment creates a condition in which the regular cells hibernate as cancer cells run amok, making you more susceptible.

Research has demonstrated that fasting 'protects regular but not cancerous cells against elevated treatment' in a paper released in 2008. It was followed up with a report showing that fasting improved the effectiveness of chemotherapy medications in the treatment of a number of cancers.

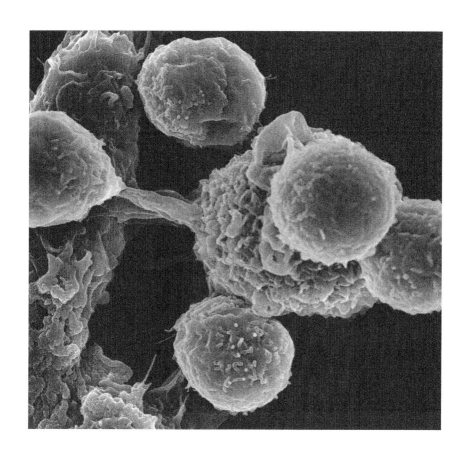

Chapter 7: The Psychological Benefits of Intermittent Fasting

The very first element you can predict from intermittent fasting is losing weight: some months more, some months less; certain weeks you'll hit a frustrating plateau, and other weeks you'll see faster gains.

If the weeks pass, you'll see that Intermittent Fasting has several beneficial side effects. There are more powerful effects, benefits, and incentives that may come into play in addition to the apparent fat loss and potential health advantages. So, indeed, you'll begin to break unhealthy eating habits. However, if you manage to fast — and feed — with vigilance, you can notice a variety of other improvements, some of which are impossible and unpredictable. For example, you might learn that you've been suffering from 'size delusion' for years, believing that the amount of food on your plate is the amount you really want and desire. Over practice, you'll actually realize you've been doing so much. So it's not just the physical burden that you'll be able to put off with intermittent fasting but also the mental exhaustion that has been tiring you for years. Read this chapter to find out what intermittent fasting can do for your brain and mental health.

7.1 Mood Regulation and Intermittent Fasting

According to Professor Mark Mattson, one of the factors people can find Intermittent Fasting pretty simple to do is its impact on BDNF. Not only does BDNF seem to shield the brain from aging and age-related mental deterioration, but it can even boost the attitude.

Many research, dating back several years, have shown that increasing BDNF levels have an antidepressant impact, initially in rodents. In one study, researchers inserted BDNF straight into the minds of rats and discovered that it has comparable results to using a normal antidepressant regularly. LQ Another study discovered that electric shock treatment, which has been shown to help people with extreme depression, seems to succeed in part because it induces the development of further BDNF.

Mark Mattson claims that BDNF levels would begin to increase within a few weeks of starting a two-day-a-week fasting regimen, reducing fear and elevating mood. He doesn't yet have enough human evidence to back up his argument, but he is conducting tests on volunteers that include, among other items, taking daily specimens of cerebrospinal fluid (the fluid that cleans the brain) to evaluate the modifications that arise during intermittent fasting. This is not a trial for the heart's weakness since it necessitates frequent spinal taps, but as Mark points out to me, several of his participants are now showing signs of cognitive improvement, so they are highly inspired. Mark is passionate about researching and promoting the effectiveness of Intermittent Fasting because he is concerned about the long-term consequences of the ongoing obesity crisis on our minds and culture. He also believes that if you are contemplating Intermittent Fasting, you can get started as soon as possible.

'The activities that arise in mind at the stage of the nerve cells and the chemicals in the nerve fibers, such modifications occur very early, perhaps decades before the topic begins to experience understanding and memory issues,' says the researcher. That is why it is essential to begin nutritional regimens early in life. At the same time, people are young or middle-aged to delay the progression of certain mechanisms in the brain and continue to be 90 with a fully functional brain. Like Mark, I believe that abstaining from food for brief amounts of time protects the human brain. This is a fascinating and rapidly developing field of science that many people would be watching with bated breath. Further than the brain, Intermittent Fasting has observable, positive results on other parts of the body, including the heart, blood profile, and cancer risk. And it's to this that we'll now transform.

7.2 Anxiety and Intermittent Fasting

Intermittent fasting's science is fascinating. You'd be shook that it can immensely help you with your anxiety and mental health in general.

Fasting encourages the production of a hormone named ghrelin, which aids in the perception of appetite in the brain. As a result, the extensively and more regularly you fast, the farther your body adjusts to the new routine. The impact of the science of skipping breakfast on brain wellbeing was explained by Yocheved Golani, a licensed Health Management professional: "Intermittent fasting is beneficial to the brain. Intermittent fasting is a method of going without food for a few hours, allowing the body to rid itself of waste such as bacteria and viruses, dead and deteriorated cells, weakened organelles (tiny molecular structures that serve various roles in our bodies), and damaged proteins.

Autophagy, or internal cleaning, allows the body to work better by making you feel more energized and clear-headed.

It slows the progression of certain illnesses, reduces the symptoms of Alzheimer's and Parkinson's disease, and prevents some of the detrimental consequences of aging.

Intermittent fasting enhances cellular renewal. The proteins and disease-fighting properties act like brain boosters, allowing us to think more quickly, have fewer fear and/or depression, and be healthier than normal. Through sensible intermittent fasting habits, we can also sleep easier and grow faster. Yes, intermittent fasting will hold you looking, feeling, and thinking younger, healthier, and wiser than your years." It takes some time. Making a change in your lifestyle, such as opting to pursue intermittent fasting, may be intimidating. It's OK to be hesitant; nevertheless, the impact these improvements have on your mind and body might be fascinating if you stay with them. Here are some of the beneficial mental health results of IF, some of which Golani only mentioned:

- The internal cleansing that your body undergoes helps the mind to function more efficiently.

- You feel more energized and clear-headed while you fast intermittently.

- IF prevents some cancers, and it often slows some of the detrimental consequences of aging.

- Intermittent fasting will help you sleep better.

- Your body receives more brain boosters due to cell regeneration, which allows one to think more clearly.

- Many that indulge in IF are less likely to be anxious or depressed.

When you make significant life improvements, it takes time for them to take place. It's crucial to keep in mind that these transitions and enhancements to your well-being won't happen overnight. Nevertheless, concentrating on yourself and the journey to a happier, stable existence is a wonderful first move toward progress.

Chapter 8: How To Start Intermittent Fasting

It's important to remember that intermittent fasting is not a diet. It is a method of eating that is timed. Intermittent fasting does not specify which foods a person can eat or avoid, unlike a dietary plan limiting their calories. While intermittent fasting has certain beneficial effects, including weight loss, it is not for everybody.

Intermittent fasting includes cycling between eating and fasting periods. People can find it difficult to eat only for a short period per day or to alternate between eating & not eating days.

People use intermittent fasting to: ease their lives, lose weight, and improve their general wellbeing, such as minimizing aging.

Fasting is usually safe for healthy, well-nourished individuals, although it may not be suitable for those with medical conditions.

The following tips are intended to assist those who are ready to begin fasting in making it as simple and successful as possible:

8.1 Determine your objectives.

An individual who begins intermittent fasting has a specific target in mind. That may be for weight loss, improved physical health, or better metabolic health. However, a person's overall objective will help them decide the right fasting approach and measure how many nutrients and calories they need.

8.2 Choose a method.

Before attempting another fasting process, a person should usually stay with one for at least a month.

When it comes to fasting for health reasons, there are four choices to remember. First, individuals should choose the plan that best fits their needs and believes they will adhere to.

There are following methods include:

1. Fasting on an alternate day

2. 5:2 method

3. Warrior Diet

4. Eat Stop Eat

5. Lean gains

1.   Fasting on alternate days

Before trying a new fasting method, a person should usually stick with one for a month or longer to see how it works for them. Also, before starting any fasting process, someone with a medical condition should consult their doctor.

When choosing a method, keep in mind that you don't have to eat a particular quantity or kind of food or skip certain foods entirely. An individual is free to eat whatever they want. However, it is smart to eat a balanced, vegetable-rich, high-fiber diet to meet wellness and weight loss targets during the feeding times.

On eating days, bingeing on unhealthy foods will damage your wellbeing. On the swift days, it's also important to drink plenty of water or other low-calorie drinks.

2.   5:2 method

To increase cholesterol, blood sugar, and weight loss, some people fast on alternating days. For example, on the 5:2 diet, a person consumes 500 - 600 calories on two non-consecutive days per week.

Some alternate-day fasting plans have a third fasting day each week. As a result, an individual consumes only the amounts of calories they burn during the day for the rest of the week. This results in a calorie deficit over time, causing the individual to lose weight.

3. Warrior Diet

The Warrior Diet, developed by Ori Hofmekler, involves eating very little for 20 hours per day. In the remaining four hours, a person fasting in this manner eats all of their normal food intakes.

Eating a whole day's worth of food in just a brief amount of time will disturb a person's stomach. This is the most intense fasting technique, and like Eat Stop Eat, it is not recommended for anyone new to fasting.

4. Eat stop eat

Eat Stop Eat is a fasting method developed by Brad Pilon that entails going without food for 24 hours twice a week. It makes no difference when or how long a person fasts. The only requirement is that fasting must be performed for at least 24 hours except on days that are not consecutive.

If you don't eat for 24 hours, you'll get sick. For those who are new to fasting, Eat Stop Eat may not be the right choice.

5.   Lean gains

Martin Berkhan founded lean gains for Olympic athletes, but it has since gained prominence among other people involved in fasting. Fasting for Lean gains is much shorter than it is for the Warrior Diet and Eat Stop Eat.

For example, males who prefer the Lean gains process will fast for sixteen hours and then eat whatever they want for the remaining 8 hours. Females fast for 14 hours and then eat whatever they want for the next 10 hours.

During the short, one must refrain from consuming any food but can consume as many non-calorie drinks as desired.

8.3 Determine the caloric needs

When fasting, there are no food limits, but calories must always be counted.

People who choose to lose weight would build a calorie deficit, which means they must consume less energy than they utilize. Many that want to gain weight would eat more calories than they use.

Several resources are available to help a person calculate their caloric requirements and determine how many calories they must consume per day to lose weight. An individual may also seek advice from a healthcare provider or a dietitian about how many calories they need.

8.4 Make a meal plan.

Making a weekly meal schedule will assist someone who is seeking to gain or lose weight. An individual trying to lose or gain weight can find that planning their meals for the day or week is beneficial.

Meal preparation does not have to be restrictive. Instead, it considers calorie consumption and ensures that the right nutrients are used in the diet. Meal prep has several advantages, including assisting with calorie counting and ensuring that an individual has the requisite ingredients on hand for preparing foods, quick dinners, and snacks.

8.5 Make the calories count.

Calories aren't all evenly distributed. Although these fasting practices do not specify how many calories a person can consume when fasting, Nutritional Facts must be considered.

In general, food with a high amount of nutrients or nutrient-dense food should be consumed. However, even if individuals do not have to avoid fast food completely, they can also eat it in moderation and concentrate on healthier alternatives to receive the most benefits.

Chapter 9: 14-day meal plan (Two weeks)

Before initiating intermittent fasting, make sure to contact the doctor. The actual procedure is easy if you have his or her approval. After that, you may use a regular approach, limiting daily eating to one six- to eight-hour period.

Fasting over more extended periods, such as 24, 36, 48, and 72 hours, is not always beneficial and risky.

Intermittent fasting takes two to four weeks for the body to adapt to eventually. So when you're getting used to the new schedule, you might feel hungry or anxious. Many who make it through the transition time, on the other hand, are more likely to adhere to the plan when they notice they are feeling healthier.

This 14-day meal plan is designed to assist you with implementing dietary improvements. The recipes are included in the meal plan so that you can adhere to your regular diet. These meal plans were designed to help you stay on track, save resources, and lose weight. The dietary details provided with each recipe can help you reduce your calorie consumption and maintain track of when and how much you should consume. In addition, shopping lists include everything you'll need for breakfast, lunch, and dinner throughout the week.

While following the intermitting fasting and adopting this 14-days meal plan, you should eat in the following pattern: -

- Breakfast at 9:00 a.m.
- Lunch at 12 noon
- Dinner around 6:00 p.m.

9.1 Week 1 Meal Plan

Monday:

- Breakfast: Kale Avocado Smoothie
- Lunch: Chicken Quesadilla Chaffle
- Dinner: Salmon Chaffles

Tuesday:

- Breakfast: Almond Butter Protein Smoothie
- Lunch: Chaffle & Chicken Lunch Plate
- Dinner: Cheesy Pork Chops and Butter

Wednesday:

- Breakfast: Keto Cream Cheese Pancakes
- Lunch: Sausage Ball Chaffle
- Dinner: Nilaga Filipino Soup

Thursday:

- Breakfast: Pumpkin Pie Keto Spiced Latte with simple

toasts

- Lunch: Simple Curry Turkey
- Dinner: Chicken Piccata

Friday:

- Breakfast: Keto Cauliflower Breakfast Waffles
- Lunch: Skillet Chinese ground Beef

- Dinner: Spicy Italian-style Meatballs

Saturday:

- Breakfast: Scrumptious Keto Breakfast Muffins
- Lunch: Chicken Breasts Ranch with Cheese
- Dinner: Cheesy Chicken Drumsticks

Sunday:

- Breakfast: Keto Egg Porridge
- Lunch: Chicken Unique Salad
- Dinner: Rich Meatloaf with Double-cheese

Week 1 Shopping List

Fruits and Vegetables

- Apples

- Avocado

- Bananas

- Basil Leaves

- Bell peppers, red

- Beet

- Blueberries

- Broccoli florets

- Carrots

- Cranberries

- Cilantro

- Cucumbers, English

- Green beans

- Garlic

- Kale

- Lemons

- Lettuce, Boston

- Limes

- Oregano

- Onions

- Pumpkin

- Roma tomatoes

- Scallions, green

- Baby Spinach

- Strawberries

- Tomato

Dairy and Dairy Alternatives

- Almond milk

- Cheese, Parmesan, low-fat

- Eggs (6 eggs)

- Coconut Cream (1/2 cup)

- Greek Yogurt

Spices and Herbs

- Black pepper, ground

- Cinnamon, ground

- Cloves, ground

- Coriander, ground

- Cumin, ground

- Curry powder

- Ginger, fresh (2-inch piece)

- Red pepper flakes

- Sesame seeds

- Sea salt

- Sunflower seeds

- Turmeric, ground

Fish and Seafood

- Salmon (6 ounces)

- Shrimp (6 ounces)

Meat and Poultry

- Beef, flank steak (1-pound)

- Lean Ground Lamb (1-pound)

- Chicken

- Turkey

- Beef, ground (1/2 pound)

Other

- Almonds

- Arrowroot starch

- Asparagus spears

- Apple cider vinegar

- Baking powder

- Brown Rice (1/2 cup)

- Chia seeds

- Chickpeas

- Coconut Flour

- Honey

- Hummus

- Stevia, liquid

- Maple syrup

- Nutmeg

- Oil, olive

- Oil, avocado

- Red boat fish Sauce

- Red lentils

- Rolled Oats

- Rosemary, fresh

- Serrano peppers

- Soya Sauce

- Unsweetened applesauce

- Vanilla protein powder

- Vanilla extract

- Vanilla essence

9.2   Week 2 Meal Plan

Monday:

- Breakfast: Keto Eggs Florentine

- Lunch: Old-made Chicken Soup

- Dinner: Lime Shrimp Bowl

Tuesday:

- Breakfast: Spinach Feta Keto Muffins

- Lunch: Cheesy Pottery Zucchini

- Dinner: Shredded Herbal Cattle

Wednesday:

- Breakfast: Keto Fluffy Coconut Flour Pancakes

- Lunch: Quick Steak Salad

- Dinner: Beef Barbacoa

Thursday:

- Breakfast: Keto Raspberry Brie Waffles

- Lunch: Mushrooms stuffed with beef and goat cheese

- Dinner: Tenderloin Pork with Northern Cabbage

Friday:

- Breakfast: Keto Festa Mexican Breakfast
- Lunch: Lettuce Wraps
- Dinner: Keto Zuppa Toscana

Saturday:

- Breakfast: Keto Breakfast Salmon Omelet
- Lunch: Saucy Steak Skirt with Broccoli
- Dinner: Bacon blue Zoodles Salad

Sunday:

- Breakfast: Keto Breakfast Souffle
- Lunch: Stuffed Squash Bowls of Spaghetti
- Dinner: Beef and Broccoli

Week 2 Shopping List

Fruits and Vegetables

- Apples
- Bananas
- Basil Leaves
- Bell peppers, red and yellow
- Beet

- Blueberries

- Broccoli florets

- Carrots

- Cabbage

- Chives

- Cranberries

- Cilantro

- Cucumbers, English

- Green beans

- Garlic

- Eggplant

- Kale

- Lemons

- Lettuce, Boston

- Limes

- Oregano

- Onions

- Pumpkin

- Roma tomatoes

- Scallions, green

- Baby Spinach

- Squash

- Strawberries

- Tomato

Dairy and Dairy Alternatives

- Almond milk

- Cheese, Parmesan, low-fat

- Eggs (6 eggs)

- Coconut Cream (1/2 cup)

- Greek Yogurt

Spices and Herbs

- Black pepper, ground

- Cinnamon, ground

- Cloves, ground

- Coriander, ground

- Cumin, ground

- Curry powder

- Ginger, fresh (2-inch piece)

- Red pepper flakes

- Sesame seeds

- Sea salt

- Sunflower seeds

- Turmeric, ground

- Thyme

Fish and Seafood

- Salmon (6 ounces)

- Shrimp (6 ounces)

Meat and Poultry

- Beef, flank steak (1-pound)

- Lean Ground Lamb (1-pound)

- Chicken

- Bacon

- Beef, ground (1/2 pound)

Other

- All-purpose Flour

- Almonds

- Arrowroot starch

- Asparagus spears

- Apple cider vinegar

- Baking powder

- Brown Rice (1/2 cup)

- Bay Leaf

- Balsamic Vinegar

- Coconut flour

- Chia seeds

- Chickpeas

- Corn

- Coconut Flour

- French Beans

- Flaxseed

- Honey

- Hummus

- Stevia, liquid

- Mushrooms

- Maple syrup

- Nutmeg

- Oil, olive
- Oil, avocado
- Pecans
- Red boat fish Sauce
- Red lentils
- Rolled Oats
- Rosemary, fresh
- Serrano peppers
- Soya Sauce
- Unsweetened applesauce
- Vanilla protein powder
- Vanilla extract
- Vanilla essence
- Zucchini

Chapter 10: Different Intermittent Fasting Plans

Apart from the above-given basic plan, you can also follow the below-mentioned meal plans as per the type of diet.

10.1 Intermediate fasting meal plan

This plan allows you to only eat for complete 18-hour fasting within 24 hours between 12 p.m. and 6 p.m.

Even if you skip breakfast, staying hydrated is still important. Always drink plenty of water. You can also use herbal tea (most specialists agree that coffee does not break quickly.) It has been shown that the catechins in tea enhance the effects of fasting by reducing Ghrelin's hunger hormone further until lunch, and you don't feel deprived.

You must make sure that your first meal is healthy enough because you have extended your fasting period for another four hours. After that, the burger of the 8-to-6 plan works fine, and with your dressage or top of an avocado, you can add more fats.

Seeds and nuts make good, high-fat snacks that can be eaten at approximately 2:30. Before taking them, natural enzymes like phytates that can contribute to digestive problems can be neutralized. Eat dinner at 5:30 p.m. as well as eight to six windows; it's a great option to have dinner in some kind of wild fish or other smooth protein springs with vegetables.

- First meal: Anything from the lunch recipes section at 12 noon.

- Snack: seeds and nuts, at 2:30 p.m.

- Second meal: Anything from the dinner recipes section, at 5:30 p.m.

10.2 Advanced: The revised 2-day meal plan

Eat clean for any five days a week for this plan. Then, two days later, limit your calories to a maximum of 700 every day. Calorie restriction offers many of the same advantages for a whole day as fasting.

You will have to make sure you get clean meats, healthy fats, vegetables, and certain fruits on non-fast days, and you can structure your meals but best for you.

You may have fewer meals or snacks during the entire day or have a moderate lunch and dinner quickly in the morning or after dinner during limited days. Concentrate once again on healthy fats, clean meats, and products.

Apps can help you record food to don't go over 700 and record your calorie intake.

10.1   ADVANCED: 5-2 MEALS.

On this plan, five days a week, you're going to eat clean, but you won't eat anything for two days a week.

You can quickly eat clean food on Monday and Thursday, for example. Food will be the same as other fasting plans these five days — healthy fats, clean meat, vegetables, and some fruit.

Remember that this plan is not intended for beginners. You should talk with your doctor before actually starting a fasting procedure, particularly if you are under medicine or have a medical problem. In addition, coffee drinkers are recommended to maintain a coffee supply in the morning and that all those who are fasting advanced stay properly hydrated.

- Monday: Fast.

- Tuesday: eat good fats, springs of clean meat, vegetables, and fruit.

- Wednesday: eat good fats, clean sources of meat, vegetables, and some fruit.

- Thursday: Fast.

- Friday: eat healthy fats; eat clean meat and vegetables.

- Saturday: eat healthy fat, clean sources of meat, fruit, and vegetables

10.2 **ADVANCED: EVERY OTHER DAY SCHEDULE OR ALTERNATE FASTING.**

Even if this plan is sophisticated, it is very straightforward.

You can eat healthy fats, clean meat, fruit, and vegetables every day, and then you can drink water, herbal tea, and a moderate quantity of black coffee or tea on your fasting days.

- Monday: eat clean meat, healthy fats, fruit, and vegetables.
- Tuesday: fast.
- Wednesday: eat good fats, clean sources of meat, vegetables, and some fruit.
- Thursday: fast.
- Friday: eat clean food, healthy fats, fruit, and vegetables.
- Saturday: fast.
- Sunday: eat clean meat sources, healthy fats, fruit, and vegetables.

You know precisely how to plan your meals when you start an intermittent fasting plan with this information in your hands. And although it may appear complicated at first, it'll feel like second nature and fit quite perfectly in your days once you get used to fasting. First, however, start working slowly and progressively to advanced plans.

It is also important to remember that if intermittent fasting does not work for you, you may have some "off" days. But, listen, if you have to eat outside your traditional window, it's all right. Just restart if you feel better.

Chapter 11: Physical Exercises To Combine With The Meal Plan

11.1 Exercise Types

Anaerobic and aerobic exercise both are necessary for good health. Physical fitness, also known as 'cardio,' is any activity that lasts for an extended time, like walking, racing, or swimming. Anaerobic exercise, such as sprinting or weight lifting, entails exerting maximum effort for a short period.

The type of exercise an individual does is likely to be influenced by the kind of intermittent fasting they choose. For example, anyone who follows the 16:8 plan will do either anaerobic or aerobic exercise during meals while not over-exerting.

If someone does alternating days and tries to work out on their fasting day, they should usually do something less intensive. However, if you plan to try intermittent fasting as an exercise, there are two things to keep in mind.

11.2 Exercise timing

While an individual can exercise while fasting, it may be easier to exercise after a meal.

11.3 Food type

It's crucial to know what to eat while exercising at various times of the day.

11.4 Pre-work-out nutrition

A pre-workout plan involves taking a meal 2-3 hours before exercise rather than only before exercising. It should be rich in refined carbs, such as whole-grain cereal or protein.

11.5 Post-work-out nutrition

A post-workout meal can contain fresh vegetables, high-quality proteins, and fats to aid recovery.

If a person has just worked out: the food they eat should be 50 to 60 percent of the calories in this circumstance and combine macronutrients.

If a person is going to work out later, their food should contain 30 to 50 percent of the food's calories and be made up of various macronutrients.

It is preferable to consult a doctor if a person has pre-existing health conditions and wishes to attempt intermittent fasting and exercise.

11.6 During intermittent fasting, light movement exercises include:

- Light activity is preferred to lying or sitting still
- Make a cup of coffee or tea when you wake up.
- Moving around the building
- Walking at a slow speed
- Vacuuming, dusting, and washing tasks
- Arrange your bed
- Yoga

11.7 Moderately intensive exercises:

- Aerobics in the water
- Cycling
- Briskly walking
- Exercise-style dances
- Hiking up a hill is a perfect way to spend your time outside.
- Playing Tennis with a friend
- Push a lawnmower

11.8 Aerobic exercises

Walking, Running, cycling, jogging, and dance activities are all healthy aerobic exercises. Aerobic fitness engages the body's broad muscles, supporting the cardiovascular system and weight loss. Work your way up to twenty minutes or more per session, 3 or 4 times per week. Be sure you can pass the "talk test," which requires you to exercise at a speed that allows you to carry on a conversation.

11.9 Exercises for strength

Lifting hand weights boosts balance and stamina, increases bone strength, lowers the risk of lower back injury, and helps you remain fit. Start with a hand weight that is comfortable to hold for eight repetitions. Then, gradually increase the number of reps until you hit a limit of 12.

11.10   Stretching

Stretching exercises are designed to maintain joint flexibility and range of motion. As a result, they frequently lower the risk of muscle aches and injuries. Stretching, relaxing the heart, and increasing endurance are all benefits of Yoga and Pilates.

11.13 Tips for staying healthy

When you've planned out your workout, keep the following safety tips in mind.

- Exercising after a meal: This will give a person the energy they need to finish a workout.

- Keeping a low-intensity exercise regimen: If a person is fasting, they might want to attempt low-intensity aerobic exercise. If exercising after meals, however, any form of exercise usually is healthy.

- Paying attention to what the body is saying: Whenever anyone begins to feel sick while exercising on IF, they can stop immediately.

- Keeping yourself hydrated: Even if you're not IF, staying hydrated during exercise is important. Since water makes up most of the human body, it is essential to replenish fluids depleted during exercise. Fasting or exercising can be riskier for specific individuals, such as diabetes or low blood pressure

Chapter 12: Breakfast Recipes

12.1 Kale Avocado Smoothie

Preparation Time- 10 minutes| Cook Time- 0 minutes| Total Time- 5 minutes| Servings-4 |Difficulty-Easy

Nutritional Value- Calories-114| Total Fat-6.7g |Carbohydrates-5g| Sugar-0.4g| Protein-10.9g

Ingredients

- Two cups of sliced new kale
- One cup of avocado
- One cup of almond unsweetened milk
- Half a cup of yogurt full-fat, simple
- Six-Seven cubes of ice
- Two spoonfuls of fresh lemon juice
- Stevia powder in oil, to eat

Instructions

- In a mixer, add spinach, avocado, and almond milk.
- Pulse several times on the ingredients.
- Add remaining ingredients and blend until smooth.
- Pour into a large bottle and instantly drink it.

12.2 Almond Butter Protein Smoothie

Preparation Time- 10 minutes| Cook Time- 0 minutes| Total Time- 10 minutes| Servings-4 |Difficulty-Easy

Nutritional Value- Calories-124| Total Fat-9g |Carbohydrates-2g| Sugar-0.5g| Protein-12.9g

Ingredients

- Two cups of unsweetened almond milk
- One cup of full-fat yogurt, simple
- Half cup of vanilla egg white protein powder
- Two cups of almond butter
- A pinch of cinnamon
- Extract of liquid stevia to taste

Instructions

- In a mixer, add the almond milk and yogurt.
- Pulse several times on the ingredients.
- Add remaining ingredients and blend until smooth.
- Pour into a large bottle and instantly drink it.

12.3 Keto Cream Cheese Pancakes

Preparation Time- 5 minutes| Cook Time- 15 minutes| Total Time- 20 minutes| Servings-4 |Difficulty-Easy

Nutritional Value- Calories-157| Total Fat-15g

|Carbohydrates-2.1g| Sugar-0.6g| Protein-17.9g

Ingredients

- Half cup of Crème cheese
- Four pieces of cooked chicken
- Four Eggs
- One teaspoon of Cinnamon
- Two tablespoons of coconut meal
- One Box of Wild stevia

Instructions

- Mix all of the ingredients until smooth.
- Prepare a medium-high non-stick saucepan or skillet with butter or coconut oil.
- Style them exactly like pancakes you always would.
- Try cooking on one side most of the time, and then flip!
- Cover with butter and maple syrup without sugar.

12.4 Pumpkin Pie Keto Spiced Latte

Preparation Time- 5 minutes| Cook Time- 15 minutes| Total Time- 20 minutes| Servings-4 |Difficulty-Easy

Nutritional Value- Calories-234| Total Fat-21g |Carbohydrates-2g| Sugar-1g| Protein-13.9g

Ingredients

- Four cups of coffee, with a solid and fresh brew
- Two cups of coconut milk
- Half cup of Kitten Puree
- Four teaspoons of Pumpkin Pie Seasoning Blend
- One teaspoon of Cinnamon Powder
- Two tablespoons of Vanilla Powder
- Two cups of Strong Whipped Cream
- Two Spoonful of Butter
- Twenty Drops Stevia Liquid

Instructions

- Cook squash, sugar, butter, and spices over medium-low heat
- Add 2 cups of strong coffee until bubbling and combine
- Remove from a burner, apply cream and stevia and merge with an immersion blender.
- Whipped cream on the tip, and enjoy.

12.5 Keto Cauliflower Breakfast Waffles

Preparation Time- 5 minutes| Cook Time- 0 minutes| Total Time- 5 minutes| Servings-4 |Difficulty-Easy

Nutritional Value- Calories-189| Total Fat-14g |Carbohydrates-5g| Sugar-0.3g| Protein-14.9g

Ingredients

- One cup of grated Mozzarella Cheese
- One cup of Raw Cauliflower
- One cup of Parmesan cheese
- One cup of Cheddar Cheese
- Four Big Eggs
- Table cubit Chives, Sliced
- One cup of onion powder
- One cup of garlic powder
- Salt and pepper as per taste
- A quarter tablespoon of red pepper flakes to fit

Instructions

- Slice the cauliflower into blooms.
- Use of a food processor to feed by grating attachment
- Add cheese, then adds eggs and spices to the grill and blend.
- Cook and toss 1/2 of the mixture into a waffle maker
- Remove from waffle
- Top with the toppings you need.

12.6 Scrumptious Keto Breakfast Muffins

Preparation Time- 10 minutes| Cook Time- 25 minutes| Total Time- 35 minutes| Servings-4 |Difficulty-Easy

Nutritional Value- Calories-211| Total Fat-15.3g |Carbohydrates-1g| Sugar-0.2g| Protein-15.9g

Ingredients

- Two medium Eggs
- One cup of Heavy Cream
- Two slices cooked Bacon (Cured, Pan-Fried, Cooked)
- Two oz. Cheddar Cheese
- Salt & Black Pepper (to taste)

Instructions

- Heat oven to 350º F.
- Whisk the eggs in a cup with sugar, salt, and pepper.
- Spread the muffin tins into pam, and fill the cups 1/2 full.
- Place one slice of crumbled bacon on top of each muffin, and then 1/2 oz. Cheese.
- Bake for about 15-20 minutes or until light brown.
- Add 1/2 oz. of cheese on each muffin and broil until the cheese has browned slightly. Enjoy it!

12.7 Keto Egg Porridge

Preparation Time- 10 minutes| Cook Time- 20 minutes| Total Time- 30 minutes| Servings-4 |Difficulty-Easy

Nutritional Value- Calories-196| Total Fat-6.8g |Carbohydrates-3g| Sugar-0.3g| Protein-14.9g

Ingredients

- Four organic free-range eggs
- One and a half cups of organic heavy cream without food additives
- Four packages of stevia Or your preferred sweetener to taste
- Four tablespoons of grass-fed butter
- A pinch of ground organic cinnamon to taste
- Berries to garnish

Instructions

- Add the whites, milk, and sweetener to a small bowl and whisk together
- Heat the butter over medium to high heat in a heavy saucepan. When the butter is warmed, raise the heat to a minimum temperature.
- Combine the egg and the milk mixture.
- Boil, blend all the time around the bottom until the mixture thickens and starts to curdle.

- When you see the first signs of curdling, quickly remove the saucepan from the sun.
- Pour the porridge into a dish to drink. Sprinkle lots of cinnamon on top and berries and serve right away.

12.8 Keto Eggs Florentine

Preparation Time- 5 minutes| Cook Time- 20 minutes| Total Time- 25 minutes| Servings-4 |Difficulty-Easy

Nutritional Value- Calories-184| Total Fat-14.3g |Carbohydrates-3.1g| Sugar-0.4g| Protein-14.9g

Ingredients

- Two cups of cleaned fresh spinach
- Four tablespoons of finely grated parmesan cheese
- Ocean salt and chili as per taste
- One cup of white vinegar
- Four Eggs

Instructions

- Cook the spinach in a healthy microwave bowl or steam until wilted
- Sprinkle with the parmesan cheese to taste and season.
- Slice bits in bite-size and put them on a tray.

- Heat a tub of boiling water, add the vinegar and stir to make a whirlpool using a wooden spoon.
- Break the egg into the middle, turn the heat, and keep covered (3-4 minutes) until set. Repeat for 2nd seed.
- Place the spinach with eggs and drink.

12.9 Spinach Feta Keto Muffins

Preparation Time- 10 minutes| Cook Time- 40 minutes| Total Time- 50 minutes| Servings-4 |Difficulty-Moderate

Nutritional Value- Calories-234| Total Fat-21.7g |Carbohydrates-4g| Sugar-0.6g| Protein-14.9g

Ingredients

- Eight eggs
- Four slices bacon, cooked
- Three cups of raw spinach
- One and a half cups of crumbled feta cheese
- One cup of cheddar cheese
- Salt and pepper to taste

Instructions

- Preheat oven to 350 degrees F.
- Wash the spinach, rinse and put in a healthy bowl for microwave use
- Microwave the spinach for 1 minute on fast.

- Re-cool back.
- Bacon has to be fried until you need it. Then, put it aside to freshen up.
- Pound the eggs together in a small mixing cup until shiny.
- Mix the crumbled feta cheese and dried cheddar cheese.
- Upon ample cooling of the spinach and bacon, add to the bowl, and blend until mixed.
- Split the mixture equally into 6 cups of muffins. Bake until the muffins are solid for 30-35 minutes.

12.10   Keto Fluffy Coconut Flour Pancakes

Preparation Time- 20 minutes| Cook Time- 0 minutes| Total Time- 20 minutes| Servings-4 |Difficulty-Easy

Nutritional Value- Calories-211| Total Fat-14.5g |Carbohydrates-2.1g| Sugar-0.6g| Protein-15.9g

Ingredients

- Two cups of coconut flour
- Two cups of granulated erythritol
- Two teaspoons of baking powder
- Two teaspoons of salt
- Six large, lightly beaten eggs
- Half cup of melted butter

- Two cups of almond milk
- Extra butter or oil for cooking
- One teaspoon vanilla extract

Instructions

- Preheat oven to 200°F.
- Beat together erythritol, coconut flour, salt, and baking powder in a bowl.
- Beat together melted butter, eggs, vanilla extract, and almond milk in another bowl.
- Combine both the prepared mixtures and mix well
- Heat a saucepan over a medium-high flame and brush it with melted butter or vegetable oil.
- Pour two tablespoons of batter onto the saucepan and spread it into circular motion making a 3 to 4-inch circle.
- Cook until the top is set around the edges and the base is golden brown.
- Flip it carefully and continue until the second side of the pancake is golden brown, then transfer it to a plate. Repeat with the rest of the batter.
- Serve warm and enjoy!

12.11   Keto Raspberry Brie Waffles

Preparation Time- 10 minutes| Cook Time- 25 minutes| Total Time- 35 minutes| Servings-4 |Difficulty-Easy

Nutritional Value- Calories-195| Total Fat-16.3g |Carbohydrates-2 g| Sugar-1g| Protein-13.9g

Ingredients

For the Waffles

- Half cup of Almond Flour
- Two tablespoons of Flaxseed Meal
- 1/3 cup of Coconut Milk
- Vanilla Extract
- One teaspoon of Baking Powder
- Two Large Eggs
- Two tablespoons of Swerve
- Seven drops of Liquid Stevia

For the Filling

- Half cup of raspberries
- Zest of half Lemon
- One tablespoon of Lemon Juice
- Two tablespoons of Butter
- One tablespoon of Swerve
- Three oz. of Double Cream Brie

Instructions

- Add all the waffle ingredients together and blend properly.
- Cook over a waffle iron instead.
- Remove from waffle iron and put brie slices over waffles.
- Melt oil in a saucepan and dissolve.
- When browned, add lemon juice/zest and raspberries.
- Let it steams until it bubbles and is jam-like.
- Set the waffle sides under a broiler until the brie is smooth and the waffle is finely crisp.
- Assemble brie waffle and raspberry compote. "Grill" in a medium-heat pan for 1-2 minutes on each side.

12.12   Keto Festa Mexican Breakfast

Preparation Time- 10 minutes| Cook Time- 15 minutes| Total Time- 25 minutes| Servings-4 |Difficulty-Easy

Nutritional Value- Calories-191| Total Fat-14.6g |Carbohydrates-2.1g| Sugar-0.2g| Protein-17.9g

Ingredients

- Four eggs, poached
- A quarter cup of chunky salsa
- 1/3 cup of cheddar cheese, shredded
- 1/3 cup of avocado, cut into chunks

- Two tablespoons of sour cream
- Two tablespoons of sliced olives
- Two tablespoons of finely chopped fresh cilantro

Instructions

- Cook the eggs using poaching.
- Steam the salsa in a microwave-protected dish.
- Put the poached eggs on the serving plate and add sauce, sour cream, olives, milk, avocado, and parsley on top.

12.13   Keto Breakfast Salmon Omelet

Preparation Time- 5 minutes| Cook Time- 10 minutes| Total Time- 15 minutes| Servings-4 |Difficulty-Easy

Nutritional Value- Calories-188| Total Fat-18.4g |Carbohydrates-2 g| Sugar-0.2g| Protein-21.9g

Ingredients

- Six eggs
- Two smoked salmon
- Six links pork sausage
- One cup of onions
- One cup of provolone cheese

Instructions

- Whisk the eggs and can them in a squash.

- Follow the traditional omelet process, adding onions, salmon, and cheese to the omelet before spinning.
- Sprinkle finished omelet with extra cheese and serve side links with sausage.

12.14   Keto Breakfast Soufflé

Preparation Time- 5 minutes| Cook Time- 15 minutes| Total Time- 20 minutes| Servings-4 |Difficulty-Easy

Nutritional Value- Calories-174| Total Fat-17.2g |Carbohydrates-2.1g| Sugar-0.3g| Protein-16.9g

Ingredients

- One cup of egg whites
- Six tablespoons of unsalted butter
- One cup of thinly sliced mushrooms
- Half medium thinly sliced tomato
- Salt and pepper to taste
- One cup crumbled fresh goat cheese or cheese of your choice

Instructions

- Preheat oven to 400º F.
- Mix egg whites with salt and pepper and whip them into small peaks.

- Warm the oil over high heat and sauté the mushrooms until tender in a healthy frying pan or cast-iron skillet.
- Put sliced tomatoes over the mushroom.
- Fold cheese easily into egg white mixture and spillover mushroom/tomato mixture.
- Put the frying pan in the oven and bake for about 8 minutes.
- Flip soufflé over the serving plate from the oven.

Chapter 13: Lunch Recipes

13.1 Chicken Quesadilla Chaffle

Preparation Time-10 minutes| Cook Time-15 minutes| Total Time- 25 minutes| Servings-4 | Difficulty-Easy

Nutritional Facts- Calories-99Cal| Total Fat-8g |Saturated Fat-0g |Cholesterol-0mg |Total Carbohydrates-4g

Ingredients

- One teaspoon of taco seasoning
- One cup of cooked and chopped chicken
- Two beaten eggs
- One cup of finely grated cheddar cheese

Instructions

- Preheat the waffle iron.
- In a medium bowl, mix the eggs, taco seasoning, and cheddar cheese. Add the chicken and combine well.
- Open the iron, lightly oil with cooking spray and pour in half of the mixture.
- Close the iron and cook until brown and crispy, 7 minutes. Remove the chaffle onto a plate and set it aside.
- Make another chaffle using the remaining mixture. Serve afterward.

13.2 Chaffle & Chicken Lunch Plate

Preparation Time-10 minutes| Cook Time-15 minutes| Total Time- 15 minutes| Servings-4 | Difficulty-Easy

Nutritional Facts- Protein-31% |Fat-66% |Carbohydrates-2%

Ingredients

- A pinch salt
- One cup of shredded jack cheese
- Two large egg

For Serving

- Salt
- Two teaspoons of garlic paste
- Two teaspoons of avocado oil
- Two chicken legs
- Pepper
- Two egg

Instructions

- Heat your square waffle-making machine and oil with cooking spray.
- Pour Chaffle batter into the skillet and cook for about 3 minutes. Put a pan over medium heat and heat the oil.

- Once the oil is hot, add chicken thigh and garlic then, cook for about 5 minutes. Flip and cook for another 3-4 minutes. Season with pepper and salt and mix well. Transfer cooked thigh to plate.
- Fry the egg in the same pan for about 1-2 minutes.
- Once chaffles are cooked, serve with a fried egg and chicken thigh. Enjoy!

13.3 Sausage Ball Chaffle

Preparation Time-5 minutes| Cook Time-10 minutes| Total Time- 15 minutes| Servings-4 | Difficulty-Easy

Nutritional Facts- Calories-245|Fat-13.4 g|Protein-19.2 g|Carbohydrates-1.1 g

Ingredients

- Four tablespoons of flour
- One cup of grated cheddar cheese
- Two eggs
- One pound of Italian sausage
- Two teaspoons of baking powder
- Half cup of grated parmesan cheese

Instructions

- In a bowl, combine Italian sausage, flour, baking powder, cheddar cheese, and egg. Make sure you kneed these ingredients well.

- Then turn on the waffle-making machine and preheat it to medium heat. Then sprinkle some parmesan cheese on the waffle-making machine and let it cook for about 30 seconds.
- Then pour the mixture on top of the cheese and close the lid of the waffle machine.
- Let the chaffle cook for about 3 to 5 minutes until it is golden brown. This way, you will have delicious chaffless ready to be eaten.

13.4 Simple Curry Turkey

Preparation Time- 10 minutes| Cook Time- 50 minutes| Total Time- 1 hour | Servings-4 |Difficulty-Hard

Nutritional Value- Calories-295| Total Fat-2.9g |Carbohydrates-0 g| Sugar-0.6g| Protein-3.1g

Ingredients

- Three teaspoons of Sesame oil
- One pound of turkey legs
- Two cloves
- One red chili pepper
- Half tablespoon of minced garlic
- Half teaspoon of ginger powder
- Turmeric powder

- One teaspoon of red curry paste
- One cup of unsweetened coconut milk
- Half cup of water
- Half cup of turkey
- Kosher salt and Black Pepper to taste

Instructions

- Heat the sesame oil in a minced pan. Attach the turkey and simmer till light brown, around seven minutes.
- Add garlic, chili pepper, curry spice, and turmeric powder—Cook 3 more minutes. Add the milk and water, and feed. Season with black pepper and oil. Cooking At moderate heat for 45 minutes.

13.5 Skillet Chinese ground beef

Preparation Time- 10 minutes| Cook Time- 20 minutes| Total Time- 30 minutes| Servings-4 |Difficulty-Easy

Nutritional Value- Calories-242| Total Fat-24g |Carbohydrates-6g| Sugar-0.6g| Protein-26.9g

Ingredients

- Two tablespoons of sesame oil
- One pound chuck
- Two shallots
- Two chopped garlic cloves

- Some cloves
- Two (1/2) "slice of ginger root, peeled and rubbed
- Two bell peppers
- Eight ounces of brown mushrooms crushed and diced
- Two tablespoons of tamari soy
- Two tablespoons of rice wine
- Four-star anise
- Himalayan salt and black pepper, to taste

Instructions

- Warm the oil in a saucepan over a medium flame. Then roast the ground chuck until it's cooked or isn't pink anymore; Reserve.
- Then in pan drippings, cook the shallot, garlic, ginger, pepper, and mushrooms. Finally, apply the rest of the ingredients and the retained beef to the saucepan. Decrease temperature to medium-low; allow it to simmer for 2 to 3 more minutes. Let it happen. Then serve.

13.6 Chicken Breasts Ranch with Cheese

Preparation Time- 5 minutes| Cook Time- 20 minutes| Total Time- 25 minutes| Servings-4 |Difficulty-Easy

Nutritional Value- Calories-295| Total Fat-3g |Carbohydrates-2g| Sugar-0.3g| Protein-19g

Ingredients

- Four Chicken breasts
- Four spoons of sugar
- Two tablespoons of salt
- One teaspoon of Garlic
- One teaspoon of cayenne pepper paste
- One teaspoon of black peppercorns, ground
- One teaspoon ranch seasoning blend
- Eight ounces of Ricotta cheese
- One cup of Monterey-Jack cheese
- Eight slices of bacon
- Half cup of minced scallions

Instructions

- Preheat your oven to 370 ° Fahrenheit Sprinkle with melted butter over the Chicken. Season the chicken with salt and garlic powder, a seasoning blend of cayenne Pepper, Black Pepper, and ranch.
- Set moderate-heat a cast-iron skillet. Boil the chicken for 3 to 5 minutes by hand. Place the chicken in a lightly greased baking dish. Add bacon and cheese. Bake for 12 minutes. Scallions on end right before
- Serve. Better hunger.

13.7 Chicken Unique Salad

Preparation Time- 5 minutes| Cook Time- 20 minutes| Total Time- 25 minutes refrigeration time excluded| Servings-4 |Difficulty-Easy

Nutritional Value- Calories-284| Total Fat-19g |Carbohydrates-3g| Sugar-0.6g| Protein-17.6g

Ingredient

- Two skinless chicken breasts
- Half cup mayonnaise
- Half cup of sour cream
- Four spoons Cottage cheese, ambient temperature
- Salt and black pepper as per taste
- Half cup of Sunflower seeds
- One avocado
- Half tablespoons of peeled and cubed Garlic
- Four spoonsful of sliced scallions

Instructions

- Place a very well-salted pot of water to a gentle simmer. Add the chicken to the hot water; turn the heat down low, and let the Chicken stay for 15 minutes.

- Remove the bowl, then; cut the chicken into pieces of bite-size. Add the rest of the products and mix them properly. Set in the fridge for at least an hour.

13.8 Saucy Steak Skirt with Broccoli

Preparation Time- 5 minutes| Cook Time- 25 minutes| Total Time- 30 minutes refrigeration time excluded| Servings-4 |Difficulty-Easy

Nutritional Value- Calories-264| Total Fat-20g |Carbohydrates-2.1g| Sugar-0.6g| Protein-18.9g

Ingredients

- Two pounds skirt steak
- Two tablespoons of butter cut into parts, room temperature
- Two pounds of broccoli
- Two cups of scallions sliced into florets
- Four cloves of garlic sliced to bits

For marinade Press

- Two teaspoons of black pepper
- Four teaspoons of red pepper
- Two teaspoons of sea salt flakes
- Two tablespoons of olive oil
- One tablespoon of tamari sauce

- One cup of Vinegar wine

Instructions

- Both components for the marinade are carefully mixed in a ceramic pot. Add the beef & allow it to remain in your fridge for 2 hours. Dissolve one spoonful of butter over strong to medium-high heat in a pan. Cook the dishes broccoli, regularly mixing for 2 minutes, till soft yet bright green, reserve.

- Melt the remaining butter tablespoon into the skillet— Cook the once warm, Scallions and garlic for about 2 minutes, before aromatic, reserve. Then grill the steak, applying a limited amount of marinade. Process till smooth brown on both levels, perhaps 10 minutes and so. Insert the stored vegetables and start cooking for several minutes or until everything is ready and heated. Excellent appetite.

13.9 Old-made Chicken Soup

Preparation Time- 10 minutes| Cook Time- 55 minutes| Total Time- 1 hour and 5 minutes| Servings- 4 |Difficulty- Hard

Nutritional Value- Calories-283| Total Fat-15.9g |Carbohydrates-2.1g| Sugar-0.6g| Protein-35.8g

Ingredients

- One Rotisserie chicken
- Six cups of water
- Two tablespoons of butter
- Two stalks of celery
- Half chopped onion
- One bay leaf
- Sea salt and Black Pepper, to taste
- One tablespoon of fresh coriander
- Two cups of kale chopped in strips

Instructions

- Fry the bone and carcasses with water over average build from a remaining chicken 15-minute heat. After which, minimize to a simmer and prepare a further 15 Minutes. Set back the Chicken and the broth.
- Tear the meat into bite-size pieces; let Everything chill enough just to eat. Melt the butter over a moderate flame in a big soup pot.
- Stir with celery and onion to the point of being delicate and citrusy. Remove bay leaves, salt, pepper, and broth and cook for 10 minutes.
- Attach the reserved Chicken, cilantro, and cabbage. Simmer an extra 10 to 11 minutes once cabbage is a Good tender appetite.

13.10   Cheesy Pottery Zucchini

Preparation Time- 10 minutes| Cook Time- 50 minutes| Total Time- 1 hour and 5 minutes| Servings-4 |Difficulty- Hard

Nutritional Value- Calories-214| Total Fat-11.7g |Carbohydrates-9g| Sugar-1g| Protein-12.9g

Ingredients

- Non-stick cooking spray
- Two cups of zucchini
- Two tablespoons leeks thinly diced
- Half teaspoon of salt
- Freshly ground black pepper
- Half teaspoon of dried basil
- Half tablespoon of dried oregano
- Half cup of cheddar cheese, grated
- A quarter cup of heavy cream
- Four tablespoons of parmesan cheese
- One tablespoon of butter

Instructions

- Preheat the oven to 370 degrees F. Grease a saucepan gently. Use a non-stick mist for cooking.
- Add one tablespoon of new garlic, hazelnuts. Place 1 cup of zucchini slices in the dish; add one spoonful of

leeks; sprinkle. Season with oil, basil, pepper, and oregano. Finish Cheddar cheese with 1/4 cup. Echo the layers once again.

- Whisk the heavy cream in a mixing dish with Parmesan, butter, and Garlic. Break this combination over the layer of zucchini and the layers of cheese.
- Position in the preheated furnace and cook to the outside for around 40 to 45 minutes till the edges are beautifully browned. Spray with chopped chives, if required.

13.11   Quick Steak Salad

Preparation Time- 5 minutes| Cook Time- 20 minutes| Total Time- 25 minutes| Servings-4 |Difficulty-Easy

Nutritional Value- Calories-200| Total Fat-17.4g |Carbohydrates-0.7g| Sugar-0.6g| Protein-24.9g

Ingredients

- Four tablespoons of olive oil
- 16- ounces flank steak, flavored with salt and pepper
- Two Cucumbers
- One cup of sliced carrots
- Two ripe avocadoes finely sliced, peeled, and trimmed
- Four Small-sized heirloom tomatoes
- Four ounces of sliced arugula

- Two tablespoons of clean baby coriander
- Six spoons of lime juice

Instructions

- Heat 1 spoonful of olive oil over medium to high heat in a cup. Prep the sides Steak, turn once or twice, for 5 minutes. Let's stay for 10 minutes, so finely slice over the grain. Place the meat over to one pot.
- Include cucumbers, shallots, avocado, tomatoes, fresh coriander, and baby arugula. Sprinkle the salad with lime juice and the remaining one tablespoon of olive oil.
- Serve cooled sufficiently, and eat!

13.12 Mushrooms stuffed with beef and goat cheese

Preparation Time- 5 minutes| Cook Time- 20 minutes| Total Time- 25 minutes| Servings-4 |Difficulty-Easy

Nutritional Value- Calories-222| Total Fat-19.2g |Carbohydrates-3g| Sugar-0.6g| Protein-28.6g

Ingredients

- 8- ounces of ground beef
- 4- ounces of ground pork
- Kosher salt and black pepper

- One cup of goat cheese
- Four tablespoons of Romano cheese crumbled, grated
- Four spoonsful of shallot, diced
- Two garlic cloves, dry
- Two teaspoons of oregano dried basil
- One teaspoon of rosemary dry
- 40- button Champignons, stems cut

Instructions

Add all ingredients in a baking pot, except perhaps the mushrooms. Then there's Stuff the mushrooms with the filling.

Bake for about 18 minutes in the oven and bake at 370 degrees Fahrenheit. Service Warm and cold. Better hunger.

13.13   Lettuce Wraps

Preparation Time- 10 minutes| Cook Time- 10 minutes| Total Time- 20 minutes| Servings-4 |Difficulty-Easy

Nutritional Value- Calories-177| Total Fat-11.2g |Carbohydrates-2.1g| Sugar-0.6g| Protein-16.9g

Ingredients

- Two tablespoons soy sauce
- One teaspoon sesame oil
- One tablespoon olive oil
- 4 ounces water chestnuts, drained and diced
- One tablespoon fresh ginger, minced
- 1/3 cup hoisin sauce
- One and a half tablespoons of rice wine vinegar
- One pound of ground chicken
- One carrot, peeled and diced
- Two teaspoons garlic, minced
- Two teaspoons fresh ground ginger
- Two small heads of Bibb or butter lettuce
- A quarter cup of sliced green onions, optional

Instructions

- Whisk together the rice wine vinegar, soy sauce, hoisin sauce, and sesame oil in a tiny cup. Set it aside.
- Clean the lettuce by rinsing it. Then, place the whole head of lettuce on a plate for quick picking, or separate the leaves and stack them.
- Brown the ground chicken in olive oil over medium heat for around 6-7 minutes. In a large mixing bowl, combine the diced carrots, garlic, ginger, and water chestnuts. Before applying the hoisin sauce mixture, stir for around a minute. To add, mix thoroughly.

Transfer to a serving bowl and eat with the lettuce leaves or heads.

13.14   Stuffed Squash Bowls of Spaghetti

Preparation Time- 10 minutes| Cook Time- 1 hour and 10 minutes| Total Time- 1 hour and 20 minutes| Servings-2 to 4 |Difficulty-Hard

Nutritional Value- Calories-266| Total Fat-9.3g |Carbohydrates-9.7g| Sugar-0.6g| Protein-12.9g

Ingredients

- Half pound spaghetti
- Squash, halved, scoop out seeds
- One teaspoon olive oil
- Half cup of mozzarella cheese, shredded
- Half cup of cream cheese
- Half cup of full-fat Greek yogurt
- Two eggs
- One garlic clove, minced
- Half teaspoon of cumin
- Half teaspoon of basil
- Half teaspoon lime
- Sea salt and black chili pepper, to taste

Instructions

- Put the half squash in a cooking skillet; drizzle the insides of each quarter squash of cooking olive oil.

- Bake in an oven and bake for 45 to 50 minutes at 370 degrees F, until its Interior spaces are easy to pierce with a fork. Now clean the spaghetti out "Noodles" with skin squash in a blending pot. Add leftover components and blend properly.

- Load each squash half cautiously with the cheese mixture. Cook at 350 degrees F for 5 to 10 minutes, till the cheese is golden brown and fizzing.

Chapter 14: Dinner Recipes

14.1 Salmon Chaffles

Preparation Time-6 minutes| Cook Time-10 minutes| Total Time- 16 minutes| Servings-4 | Difficulty- Easy

Nutritional Facts- Carbohydrates-3 g|Fat-10 g|Protein-5 g|Calories-201

Ingredients

- One cup of shredded mozzarella cheese
- Two large eggs
- Two tablespoons of cream cheese
- Two tablespoons of everything bagel seasoning
- Four slices of salmon

Instructions

- Turn on the waffle-making machine to heat and oil it with cooking spray.
- Beat egg in a bowl, and then add half a cup of mozzarella.
- Introduce half of the mixture into the waffle-making machine and cook for 4 minutes.
- Remove and repeat with the remaining mixture.
- Let chaffles cool, then spread cream cheese, sprinkle with seasoning, and top with salmon.

14.2 Cheesy Pork Chops and Butter

Preparation Time- 5 minutes| Cook Time- 25 minutes| Total Time- 30 minutes| Servings-4 |Difficulty-Easy

Nutritional Value- Calories-302| Total Fat-23g |Carbohydrates-2g| Sugar-0.5g| Protein-27.9g

Ingredients

- One cup of white onion at room temperature
- One pound of grilled pork chops
- Two tablespoons of ground parsley flakes
- Salt and ground black pepper
- One cup of Swiss cheese to taste, shredded

Instructions

- Heat 1/4 of the stick butter over a moderate flame in a pan. Stir in the onions, then and the champignons are soft till the onions become yellow, then spiced around 5 minutes. Reserve. Then melt the leftover 1/4 of the stick of butter and cook pork before mildly brown on both parts for about ten minutes.
- Insert the combination of onions, parsley, salt, and chili pepper. Last but not least, top with cheese. Let it cook over medium-low heat till the cheese melts. Serve right away, and enjoy!

14.3 Nilaga Filipino Soup

Preparation Time- 5 minutes| Cook Time- 45 minutes| Total Time- 50 minutes| Servings-4 |Difficulty-Moderate

Nutritional Value- Calories-298| Total Fat-24.7g |Carbohydrates-2.1g| Sugar-0.6g| Protein-29.8g

Ingredients

- Two teaspoons of butter
- Two pounds of pork ribs, boneless
- Two shallots thinly sliced
- Four garlic cloves, chopped
- Two (1/2) "slice of fresh ginger
- Two tablespoons patis (fish sauce)
- Two cups of fresh tomatoes,
- Two cups of pureed "Corn."
- Two cups of chopped cauliflower
- Ocean salt and green chili pepper, to taste

Instructions

- Melt the butter over moderate to high heat into a bowl. Warm the pork ribs on both of them instead of Sides for 5-6 minutes. Stir in shallot, garlic, and ginger; cook for 3 minutes. Add the Other ingredients.
- Let it cook for 30 to 35 minutes, sealed. Ladle, and serve in separate pots.

14.4 Chicken Piccata

Preparation Time- 15 minutes| Cook Time- 15 minutes| Total Time- 30 minutes| Servings-4 |Difficulty-Easy

Nutritional Value- Calories-451| Total Fat-29g |Carbohydrates-6g| Sugar-2g| Protein-40g

Ingredients

- One onion small
- One tablespoon of garlic minced
- Half lemon juiced (about two tablespoons)
- Three tablespoons of butter
- Four chicken breasts pounded to 1/4" thickness (2lbs)
- Ten sun-dried tomatoes cut into strips
- One and a half cups of chicken broth
- A quarter cup of capers rinsed
- 1/3 cup of heavy cream
- Four tablespoons of olive oil for frying
- Salt & pepper

Instructions

- Season the breasts with salt and pepper, then fry them in olive oil over medium-high heat on both sides until golden and cooked through (about 5-8 minutes on each side.) Remove the chicken from the pan and put it aside.

- Add the sun-dried tomatoes, onion, and garlic to the same skillet. Cook for 1-2 minutes until lightly browned, then whisk in the lemon juice, chicken broth, and capers, picking up any bits from the bottom of the plate. Allow the sauce to decrease in size by about half over medium-low heat for 10-15 minutes.

- Remove the sauce from the heat until it has thickened and whisk in the butter until it has melted, then add the cream. Return to the heat for around 30 seconds, then withdraw from the heat entirely. Serve with the chicken breasts coated in gravy.

14.5 Spicy Italian-style Meatballs

Preparation Time- 10 minutes| Cook Time- 20 minutes| Total Time- 30 minutes| Servings-4 |Difficulty-Easy

Nutritional Value- Calories-334| Total Fat-29g |Carbohydrates-5g| Sugar-1g| Protein-31g

Ingredients

For Sauce

- 6- ounces Asiago cheese
- One cup of mayonnaise
- Two chili peppers grind
- Two teaspoons of yellow mustard minced
- Two teaspoons of Italian parsley

- One teaspoon of red mustard
- Pepper flakes
- One teaspoon of sea salt ground
- One teaspoon of black pepper

For Meatballs

- One pound of beef
- Two eggs
- Two spoonfuls of olive oil

Instructions

- Integrate the cheese, mayo, curry, mustard, parsley, red pepper flakes, chili peppers, salt, and black pepper.
- Stir beef and egg in the ground then. Shake well to mix. Form a combination of meatballs. Then fire up the oil over a low flame in a pan.
- Cook the once hot, Meatballs on either flank for 2-3 minutes. Serve, and have fun!

14.6 Cheesy Chicken Drum Sticks

Preparation Time- 5 minutes| Cook Time- 20 minutes| Total Time- 25 minutes| Servings-4 |Difficulty-Easy

Nutritional Value- Calories-301| Total Fat-27.9g |Carbohydrates-2g| Sugar-0.6g| Protein-23.7g

Ingredients

- Four Chicken drumsticks
- One cup of tomato stock
- One cup of peanut butter
- Cream cheese
- Two cups of baby spinach
- Sea salt and black pepper for taste
- One teaspoon of shallot
- One teaspoon of garlic powder
- One cup of Asiago cheese

Instructions

- Warm up the oil over moderately high heat in an oven. Prep instead the Chicken for Seven Minutes, changing from time to time; reserve.
- Put in the broth; add the spinach and cream cheese; simmer until the spinach has withered. Add the chicken back to the saucepan. Remove seasonings and Asiago cheese; fry just until cooked, About 4 minutes. Serve right away.

14.7 Rich Meatloaf with double-cheese

Preparation Time- 10 minutes| Cook Time- 55 minutes| Total Time- 1 hour 5 minutes| Servings-4|Difficulty-Hard

Nutritional Value- Calories-332| Total Fat-29.6g |Carbohydrates-4g| Sugar-1g| Protein-31.8g

Ingredients

- Two tablespoons of sunflower oil
- Half cup of onions
- Two cloves of garlic, chopped
- One bell chopped pepper, seeded
- One jalapeno pepper, seeded, chopped
- A quarter-pound of bacon ground beef
- Half cup of Swiss cheese, diced
- Half cup of grated Parmesan cheese
- One egg whisked
- One teaspoon oyster sauce
- Sea salt and ground black pepper
- One teaspoon of Dijon mustard to taste
- One ripe tomato, pureed

Instructions

- Preheat your oven to 390 ° Fahrenheit. Brush a cooking pan with thin grease a non-stick mist for cooking. Steam the oil in a saucepan over a low flame. Stir in the onions, garlic, and Peppers once spicy and soft, around 5 minutes.
- Integrate the ground beef, bacon, cheese, and egg, in a blending pot, sauce of oysters, butter, and black

pepper. Shape the solution into a saucepan, place it in the frying pan, and scatter the pureed tomato and mustard combination up on top.

- Cover the dish with foil, then bake in the preheated oven for 50 minutes.

14.8 Lime Shrimp Bowl

Preparation Time- 10 minutes| Cook Time- 20 minutes| Total Time- 30 minutes| Servings-4 |Difficulty-Easy

Nutritional Value- Calories-275| Total Fat-22.5g |Carbohydrates-2.1g| Sugar-0.6g| Protein-21.7g

Ingredients

- Salt and black pepper to taste
- Half teaspoon of chili powder
- A quarter teaspoon of garlic powder
- A quarter teaspoon of smoked paprika
- 2-3 bell peppers, thinly sliced
- One lb. raw medium shrimp peeled, deveined, and tails removed
- One tablespoon chipotle pepper in adobo sauce, finely minced
- A quarter teaspoon of cumin
- A teaspoon of onion powder
- Zest and juice of one lime

- One onion, thinly sliced
- One tablespoon of butter
- One tablespoon of avocado or olive oil divided

For serving

- Fresh cilantro
- Avocado slices or guacamole
- Cauliflower rice
- Lime wedges

Instructions

- Combine the shrimp, black pepper, salt, paprika, chipotle peppers, chili powder, cumin, onion powder, garlic powder, and lime in a medium mixing cup. Set it aside.
- Cut the peppers and onions into thin slices.
- Cook onions and peppers in 1 tablespoon oil for 4-5 minutes, stirring often, or until crisp-tender. Place on a tray. As required, wipe down the pan.
- In the same pan, melt the butter and heat the remaining oil over medium heat. Sear shrimp in batches for 2-3 minutes a hand, working in batches. Transfer to a plate and repeat with the remaining shrimp, adding more oil and butter as required. When all of the shrimp is finished, return everything to the plate, even the peppers, and toss them gently until

heated through—season with a squeeze of lime and salt and pepper to taste.

- Serve with lime wedges, cilantro, and avocado, if needed, over-cooked cauliflower rice.

14.9 Shredded Herbal Cattle

Preparation Time- 5 minutes| Cook Time- 15 minutes| Total Time- 20 minutes| Servings-4 |Difficulty-Easy

Nutritional Value- Calories-294| Total Fat-21.6g |Carbohydrates-2.1g| Sugar-0.4g| Protein-27.8g

Ingredients

- Two tablespoons of olive oil
- Two pounds leg of lamb, 1/4 cut into strips (beef)
- Four tablespoons of rice wine
- One cup of beef bone broth
- Table salt and ground black pepper
- Four spoonsful of new chives, finely chopped
- Four Chipotle peppers in adobo sauce
- Three garlic cloves, chopped
- Four medium shaped chipotles, crushed
- Two mature tomatoes, peeled and pureed
- Two yellow onions, chopped
- Half tablespoon of chopped fresh Mustard and Parsley
- Two cups of dried basil

- Two cups of dried marjoram

Instructions

- Warm up the oil over medium to high warm in an oven. Sear beef for six to seven minutes, Continuously Boiling. Work in loads.
- Add the rest, heat to moderate-low, and allow to cook for forty minutes.
- Tear the beef, then eat.

14.10   Beef Barbacoa

Preparation Time- 10 minutes| Cook Time- 4 hours | Total Time- 4 hours 10 minutes| Servings-4 |Difficulty-Hard

Nutritional Value- Calories-242| Total Fat-11g |Carbohydrates-2g| Sugar-0.3g| Protein-32g

Ingredients

- Three cloves Garlic (minced)
- One teaspoon of cumin
- Two whole Bay leaf
- Two medium chipotle chiles in adobo
- One tablespoon of dried oregano
- Half teaspoon of ground cloves
- A quarter cup of Beef broth

- One tablespoon of Lime juice
- Half teaspoon of Black pepper
- One and a half lb. chuck roast or Beef brisket (cut into 2-inch chunks)
- One tablespoon of Apple cider vinegar
- One teaspoon of Sea salt

Instructions

- In a mixer, combine everything except the bay leaves and beef. Puree until entirely smooth.
- In a slow cooker, position the beef pieces. On top, pour the blended smooth mixture. Then add the bay leaves.
- Cook on high for four to six hours or low for eight to ten hours, or until the beef is soft.
- Eliminate the bay leaves. Using forks, shred the meat and add it to the juices. Cover it and set it aside for around five to ten minutes to let the beef absorb more flavor.
- Then, serve.

14.11   Tenderloin   Pork   with   Northern   Cabbage

Preparation Time- 5 minutes| Cook Time- 25 minutes| Total Time- 30 minutes| Servings-4 |Difficulty-Easy

Nutritional Value- Calories-301| Total Fat-24.8g |Carbohydrates-2.1g| Sugar-0.6g| Protein-32.7g

Ingredients

For the Pork tenderloin

- One pound of cabbage cut into strips
- One pound of pork
- Cracked black chili pepper
- One teaspoon of granulated Celtic sea salt
- Half teaspoon of ginger
- Two tablespoons of lard, room temperature
- One cup of vegetable broth
- Four tablespoons of Sherry vinegar
- One tablespoon of mustard seeds
- Scottish sea salt, to taste
- One teaspoon of green peppercorns

Instructions

- Season the pork with salt, black chili pepper, garlic, ginger powder, and sage. Burn the lard over medium heat into a saucepan.
- Caramelize through the pork for 7 to 8 minutes, starting to turn off frequently. Bring the pick, broth, sherry in a bowl heated up over moderate flame and the mustard seeds over high temperature to simmer.

Season with salt and black peppercorns; boil, stirring at frequent intervals, till cabbage is tender, for about 12 minutes; do not reheat.

- Serve the pork over the cabbage and enjoy!

14.12 Keto Zuppa Toscana

Preparation Time- 10 minutes| Cook Time- 4 hours| Total Time- 4 hours 10 minutes| Servings-4 |Difficulty-Hard

Nutritional Value- Calories-215| Total Fat-16.2g |Carbohydrates-6.4g| Sugar-3.4g| Protein-10.1g

Ingredients

- One tablespoon of oil
- Two garlic cloves, minced
- One large cauliflower head, diced into small florets
- A quarter teaspoon of crushed red pepper flakes
- Half lb. mild or hot ground Italian sausage
- A quarter cup of finely diced onion or one medium onion
- 18 oz chicken or vegetable stock
- Two cups of chopped kale
- One teaspoon of salt
- Half cup of heavy cream
- Half teaspoon of pepper

Instructions

- In a skillet over medium heat, brown the ground sausage until done.
- Remove the sausage with a slotted spoon and put it in a 6-quart slow cooker. Remove the grease and throw it out.
- In the same pan, heat the oil and cook the onions for 3-4 minutes or until translucent.
- In a slow cooker, combine the onions, cauliflower florets, chicken or vegetable stock, kale, salt, crushed red pepper flakes, and pepper. Mix so it is well blended.
- Cook for 4 hours on extreme or 8 hours on average.
- Mix in the heavy cream, so it is well mixed.

14.13 Beef and Broccoli

Preparation Time- 15 minutes| Cook Time- 30 minutes| Total Time- 45 minutes| Servings-4 |Difficulty-Moderate

Nutritional Value- Calories-255| Total Fat-11.8g |Carbohydrates-9.2g| Sugar-1.6g| Protein-28.2g

Ingredients

- Two pieces of finely chopped ginger
- Two to three minced cloves of garlic
- Two heads of broccoli broken into florets

- One lb. beef (sirloin, skirt steak, or flank steak)
- Olive oil or clarified butter (Ghee)
- Sesame seeds
- Chopped scallions

Marinade & Stir Fry Sauce

- One tablespoon and two and a half teaspoon of sesame oil
- Half teaspoon of sea salt
- Three minced garlic cloves
- Four tablespoons of coconut aminos
- One tablespoon of red boat fish sauce
- One tablespoon of freshly grated ginger
- Half teaspoon of black pepper (divided)
- A quarter teaspoon of crushed red pepper
- A quarter teaspoon of baking soda

Instructions

- Combine a half teaspoon of sea salt, two tablespoons of coconut aminos, one tablespoon of sesame oil, a quarter teaspoon of baking soda in a bowl to make the marinade.
- Combine two tablespoons of coconut aminos, one tablespoon red boat fish sauce, two teaspoons sesame oil, and pepper in a different bowl to make stir fry sauce.

- Cut the beef into quarter-inch thin slices and put it in the marinade for at least 15 minutes
- Break the broccoli into small pieces. Cover it in a microwave-safe dish with two teaspoons of water.
- Microwave for 2-3 minutes, or until it is soft then, set it aside.
- Heat one tablespoon olive oil or clarified butter (ghee) in a saucepan or wok over medium-high flame. Add in the garlic, ginger, and salt and stir for around 15 seconds.
- Raise the heat to the extreme and stir in the marinated beef. Cook for around 2 minutes, flip after the side is cooked for two to three minutes.
- Pour in the sauce. Stir-fry for 1 minute. Then add in the broccoli.
- Cook for another 30 seconds, then transfer to a plate and serve.

14.14 Bacon bleu zoodles salad

Preparation Time- 10 minutes| Cook Time- 0 minutes| Total Time- 10 minutes| Servings-4 |Difficulty-Easy

Nutritional Fact-Calories 509-kcal| Proteins-33g| Carbohydrates-9g| Cholesterol-0g | Fat-38g

Ingredients

- One cup of bleu cheese crumbled
- Eight cups of zucchini noodles
- One cup of bacon, crumbled
- One cup of spinach
- One cup of blue cheese dressing
- Pepper to taste

Instructions

- In a large mixing bowl, mix all the ingredients except zucchini noodles together.
- Serve with zucchini noodles.

Conclusion

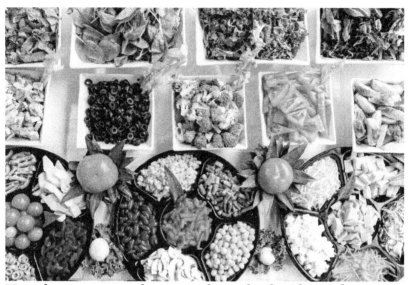

Not that you are done reading the book. Welcome to the fasting community. Fasting is, in effect, the world's oldest cure-all. "Instead of drugs, fast for a day," said Hippocrates, the founder of medicine. Furthermore, all mammals, except for current humans, naturally flee when ill or wounded. Fasting's therapeutic ability has been recognized for a long time. Still, it wasn't until recently that scientists in the fields of exercise, hygiene, diet, and healing had the scientific evidence to back it up. We published this book to reintroduce fasting as a curing mechanism, a weight loss aid, and a muscle builder, among other things. If you want to lose a few pounds, cure cancer, combat aging, or increase fertility, fasting will provide you with all of these benefits, whether you want them or not. The advantages are immense and unavoidable.

What you need is an open mind to get started. Many of the material you'll find in this book goes against popular belief. Fasting is also problematic, and the bulk of citizens aren't on board with it. "Whenever you see yourself on the field of the majority, it's time to stop and think," Mark Twain said. Think about this book as a fasting guide. Take what you want from it; you don't have to read it all the way through because you want a detailed understanding of the topic. We really don't want you to memorize something. When you've found what you're looking for, you should put this book on your shelf and pull it out if you need a refresher.

You may begin reading Chapter 1, work your way to the end, or use the Table of Contents or index to find a subject that interests you. You may choose to read only the chapters or parts of the book that concern you. Regardless, this book wishes you success in your fasting lifestyle transition, regardless of what you hear. Fasting is a straightforward term. Fasting is described as not eating for a period of time. For a bit, Despite the fact that it might seem to be counterintuitive, it is without question a very healthy and sound health method. It is, in effect, beneficial to your mind, body, and soul. You may have read that going without food is a poor thing because it slows the metabolism and causes weight gain. Ok, you've misheard. Fasting is not only beneficial to your body, but it is also possibly the healthiest thing you can do for yourself.

Fasting succeeds, and it is difficult. To be precise, it's a short-term deprivation. In the end, any diet that claims to be superior because it isn't founded on starvation is not superior at all but certainly inferior. Every diet that claims you should "eat whatever you like as long as you..." or "feed as much as you can as long as you..." is a load of garbage that should be avoided right away. Fasting will improve your health and appearance. Fasting causes the body to spontaneously tap into accumulated body fat for energy, which is severely hindered by repeatedly feeding during the day. Fasting has been shown in studies to significantly improve lipolysis, which is a fancy word for fat burning. In addition, below are a number of the health benefits that fasting will have.

Fasting is mildly stimulatory since it raises the normal adrenal reaction, which boosts your capacity. In layman's terms, that suggests that when you're fasting, your morale will rise, and your focus will boost. Fasting increases immunity and stimulates the body to detoxify itself, which helps you fight illness spontaneously. Your body purges toxic, weakened, and infected cells while fasting while still encouraging the development of new healthy cells. Eating has an aging impact on the body, largely due to insulin, the body's main food transport and blood sugar balancing hormone. Insulin is produced by your pancreas when you feed. And consuming too fast or too much has the side effect of hastening the biological aging period. Fasting slows down the aging process by lowering insulin levels. Fasting and workout potentiate each other's beneficial effects, suggesting they enhance each other's positive effects. Exercising when fasted will help you burn more calories, gain more energy, and develop muscle more effectively. Fasting has many advantages, and there is no excuse why you cannot fast on a daily basis. Fasting is, in effect, the world's oldest curing tool. Except for humans, all creatures naturally fast when ill or injured.

To conclude, many serious health problems, such as inflammation, Type-2 diabetes, and hypertension, have been known to be helped by fasting. Fasting, on the other hand, might not be enough for everybody right away. Therefore, visit your physician before beginning some fasting regimen.

If you have some health concerns that you believe could be exacerbated by fasting, talk to the doctor about it. Also, feel free to carry this book to your next appointment to review the different fasting choices with your doctor, so he or she can assist you in determining if fasting is correct for you and, if so, may fasting path is better for you.

DID YOU LIKE THIS BOOK?

If Your Answer Is Yes, I Invite You To Leave A Review on Amazon.com And Send Me A Screenshot Of It To Our Email info@suzannenewtonhealthycooking.com .

You Will Receive As A Gift A Cook-ebook pdf

Of The Ketogenic Diet with Over 650 Recipes.

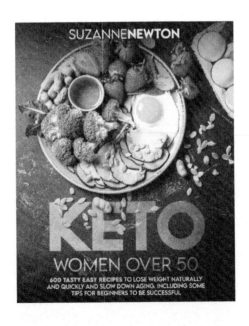

You can find suggestions, tips, tricks, and many recipes too on our website:

https://www.suzannenewtonhealthycooking.com

Printed in Great Britain
by Amazon

66811630R00119